Cultivating a
Sustainable Core

T0385217

of related interest

Integrative Rehabilitation Practice
The Foundations of Whole-Person Care for Health Professionals
Edited by Matt Erb and Arlene A. Schmid
ISBN 978 1 78775 150 7
eISBN 978 1 78775 151 4

Yoga and Science in Pain Care
Treating the Person in Pain
Edited by Neil Pearson, Shelly Prosko and Marlysa Sullivan
Foreword by Timothy McCall
ISBN 978 1 84819 397 0
eISBN 978 0 85701 354 5

Pelvic Rehabilitation
The Manual Therapy and Exercise Guide Across the Lifespan
Maureen Mason
Foreword by Ginger Garner
Illustrations by Bruce Hogarth
ISBN 978 1 91342 609 5
eISBN 978 1 91342 610 1

Pelvic Yoga Therapy for the Whole Woman
A Professional Guide
Cheri Dostal Ryba
Foreword by Shelly Prosko
Illustrations by Eve Andry
ISBN 978 1 78775 664 9
eISBN 978 1 78775 665 6

CULTIVATING A SUSTAINABLE CORE

A Framework Integrating Body, Mind, and
Breath into Musculoskeletal Rehabilitation

LIZ GILLEM DUNCANSON

Illustrations by Masha Pimas

Foreword by Shelly Prosko

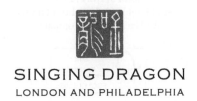

SINGING DRAGON

LONDON AND PHILADELPHIA

First published in Great Britain in 2023 by Singing Dragon,
an imprint of Jessica Kingsley Publishers
Part of John Murray Press

1

A CIP catalogue record for this title is available from the
British Library and the Library of Congress

ISBN 978 1 78775 420 1
eISBN 978 1 78775 421 8

Printed and bound in Great Britain by TJ Books Limited

Jessica Kingsley Publishers' policy is to use papers that are natural,
renewable and recyclable products and made from wood grown in
sustainable forests. The logging and manufacturing processes are expected
to conform to the environmental regulations of the country of origin.

Jessica Kingsley Publishers
Carmelite House
50 Victoria Embankment
London EC4Y 0DZ

www.singingdragon.com

John Murray Press
Part of Hodder & Stoughton Limited
An Hachette UK Company

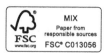

MIX
Paper from
responsible sources
FSC
www.fsc.org   FSC® C013056

For Jakob

Contents

Part II: The Sustainable Core

Part III: Practices

Foreword

It is exciting, meaningful, and rewarding to build bridges between different health care paradigms. It also brings many challenges, barriers, and frustrations. I can attest to this as a physiotherapist and yoga therapist who has focused on honing and teaching the craft of blending two related yet vastly different rehabilitation approaches throughout my entire career. I chose to be a bridgebuilder in health care over 25 years ago not because it was exciting, but because it was and continues to be invaluable and necessary for optimal evidence-informed rehabilitation.

One of my experiences as a young physiotherapist was working in an outpatient orthopedic clinic where one clinician would treat over 20 patients per day. At worst, each patient was treated as a body part. At best, the therapist would attempt to treat the whole body, but would do so within the paradigm of the "body as a machine," without consideration of any other aspect of the person's existence. Yet, we know that a person's entire physiology, along with their thoughts, beliefs, expectations, emotions, relationships with self and others (including the therapist), and sociocultural factors, all influence pain, movement, recovery, and functional outcomes. Long-time integrative bridgebuilding practitioners such as Liz, myself, and our colleagues have experienced the immense value of a whole-person (biopsychosocial-spiritual) approach and understand the urgency in implementing it more widely into musculoskeletal rehabilitation.

It's not only a few of us spouting this narrative. As David Nicholls, Associate Professor in the School of Clinical Sciences at Auckland

University of Technology, stated in his 2017 publication *The End of Physiotherapy*, "If we continue to practice physiotherapy in the manner that has seemingly worked so well for us in the past, we will become increasingly obsolete in the future. The evidence is all around us."[1] We have undeniable and growing scientific evidence that can no longer be ignored that shows our bodies do *not* function as machines.

Nicholls goes on to say that although we are being told that we need to find new ways to think and offer therapy beyond the idea of body-as-machine, we are not being shown how to do it. Indeed, even when the biopsychosocial-spiritual model is mentioned in educational settings, it is often only taught conceptually. It is challenging to translate the knowledge into practice due to its complexity.

However, in this book, Liz offers us a tangible way in. She provides an expanded and pragmatic framework of the core as a jump-off point to start this much-needed biopsychosocial-spiritual integration. She delivers an accessible and easy-to-follow guide from which to assess and serve the person in front of us. She successfully does this through the lens of and within the scope of a physical therapist, bridging her other disciplines and experiences as a dancer, musician, strength and conditioning coach, athletic trainer, and yoga therapist. Liz once explained to me how she felt her professional credentials were limiting, as they encouraged her to stay in a box—each within their own silos. She desperately needed to break through those labels of each professional identity that were restricting her creativity and her patients' potential for recovery.

Liz figured out a way to blend her knowledge, experience, skills, and wide-ranging perspectives from a mix of various fields for a more creative approach. This in turn offers more options, increasing the ability to provide individualized patient-centered care. This book is a brilliant foundational start and the reader is encouraged to continue ongoing learning about whole-person care, as no one book or person can possibly cover this comprehensive topic.

We are fortunate that Liz has decided to share her unique work; and she shares with humility. Humility is essential in science and in yoga. Without it, we risk being attached to beliefs, ideas, or practices that may limit our own learning and growth, therefore risk limiting our clients' potential and possibilities for recovery and resilience. With too much of it, we may simply avoid sharing our ideas or risk not being confident in our work, which can influence the therapeutic relationship and outcomes. Or we may freeze and fear the exploration, creativity, and courage required as a clinician. Liz embodies this humble confidence, which you will feel as you read this book.

I shared a very poignant moment in my life with Liz as she was supporting me through a challenging time. Her capacity to be fully present and hold a gracious space was healing in and of itself. I believe her remarkable gifts of compassionate listening, observing, and creating a safe space have influenced her work and this book that she shares with you today. This includes listening to and learning from the thousands of patients she has worked with, the current science, yoga, her various teachers, and her own experiences from decades of personal practice. She then organized her ideas and practices and translated her insights onto these following pages.

Whether you are a rehabilitation professional, movement educator, or a person interested in novel ways to be in your body, *Cultivating a Sustainable Core* will be an enriching learning experience for your body, mind, and spirit.

Shelly Prosko, PT, C-IAYT
Physiotherapist, yoga therapist, educator
Co-editor/author: Yoga and Science in Pain Care:
Treating the Person in Pain
www.physioyoga.ca

Disclaimer

The information contained in this book is not intended to replace the services of trained medical professionals or to be a substitute for medical advice. You are advised to consult a doctor on any matters relating to your health, and in particular on any matters that may require diagnosis or medical attention.

Note on text: A basic anatomy background is assumed.

Acknowledgments

Deepest bows of gratitude to the origins of yoga. Heartfelt thanks to my teachers: H. T. Payne, Glen Barker, Rebecca Cheema, Casey Chaney, Michael Reed Gach, Nicole Anami Becker, Debbie Gilman, Ginger Garner, Dana Damara, Matthew Taylor, Tianna Meriage-Reiter, and Sky Hegedus.

I am ever so grateful for connection. Shelly Prosko, thank you for bringing me to Maddy of Singing Dragon to listen to the pitch at the IAYT conference at Newport Beach, California in 2019. Thank you Sarah, Maddy, Victoria, and *everyone* at Singing Dragon for supporting my voice and vision and publishing this book. To Christine Koth for connecting me with Masha Pimas, the amazing illustrator! Masha, thanks for sticking with me through the global shifts and working together to help turn my brain visions into two-dimensional drawings.

Thank you to the generous people who joined the book club and helped edit drafts: Linda Wroth, Betsy Daley, Marilyn Warring, Julia Silbergeld, Robert Johnson, Harris Masket, Shari Ser, Anthony Parker, Bob Berring, Liz Williams, Lisa Vonnegut, Robert Farber, Meredith Bell, Robin Slovak, Mary Bunzel, and Mariam King. Sincere gratitude to Jason Hardage for the deluge of last-minute journal article requests! Speaking of last minute, a special bow must go to Nina Krebs who arrived into my life, ready to help, just when I asked the Universe.

Many thanks to the licensed health care providers, fitness professionals, and scientists who endured the peer-review presentation and contributed constructive feedback: Amy Selinger, Amy Day, Liz Williams, Natalie Russel, Shari Ser, Betsy Shandalov, Pam Butterfield, Betsey Noth, and Jonathan Ingersoll. Extra love sent to Tianna Meriage-Reiter for holding space and being there for me every step of this process. Special, compassionate cheers to Shelly Prosko, again for connection, and for keeping me academically honest and up to date.

Thank you to my friends, family, clients, subscribers, and therapists who have been hearing (and really listening—Sirena Masket!) about this book for the past decade. A special nod to Jhoey, Vik, and Taylor, the owners of Contra Costa Coffee, for keeping my cup full and the community safe during the pandemic shutdowns.

And to Dan—the love of my life, my partner and life-administrator. Thank you for your physical, mental, and spiritual support. Our family would not have survived the birth of this book without you.

Namaste,
Liz

Preface

Over the years, clients have asked me why no other practitioner has been able to help them the way I have. Honestly, the answer is multifactorial. Some of it has to do with the convergence of my healing paths and educational journey. I tell clients that they landed in my studio at exactly the right time for them in their journey and that they were simply ready for the next step. This book is the evidence-based support for why I combine yoga with sports medicine to help clients with musculoskeletal rehabilitation.

Please allow me to introduce myself: I am Liz, a white woman in my late 40s living in Northern California with my partner, our young son, and dog. We recently moved to suburbia into my childhood home to help care for my elderly mother. Before the global shutdown in 2020, we lived (sans Grandma) in a more urban bungalow with a private studio in the back, where I was fortunate to see private physical therapy clients for over a decade.

I love my job, and working from home was ideal when we were raising a baby and puppy. But as the practice grew, the clunky side gate, steps to enter, lack of a storefront, and the comings and goings of clients in the backyard began to hinder the business's natural pace. My schedule was full and clients often asked me to clone myself.

Once clients start to shift their awareness, they often ask me to share my secrets. "Why hasn't anyone told me this before?" they'd ask during a session. The thing is, none of this information is secret, but my academic and professional journey has led to a distillation of combined techniques from several professions. I overtly blend basic Eastern philosophies (mainly yoga, some Traditional Chinese Medicine, and Tibetan Buddhism) into my lifestyle, and that practice spills into my Western medicine physical therapy practice. Early in my career, I recall whispering to clients "This yoga stuff really works!" and explaining that "One day, the medical field will figure out how to prove it. In the meantime, let's figure out why you keep hurting yourself." That time has come. We *are* beginning to develop a greater understanding of why yoga works. This book is my attempt to demonstrate to allopathic practitioners that these methods are supported by the literature.

How can my treatment be so simple and reductionist? This book explains why I organize and reduce sessions to the five concepts of alignment, core muscle coordination, breath, awareness of self, and subtle energy. This book does not provide you with a branded "method." As an adult, I still approach life with a student's mind. Life learning is a spiral, and there are many entry points and layers of information. This is one of many possible entry or jumping-off points into this information. This book provides a look into the blend of my creative and clinical thought process. I hope that you and other practitioners find it helpful to incorporate the research and methods in your own therapy and healing practices.

My Journey

As a child, I was exposed to musical theater, dance, and percussion. I am grateful for the privilege of amazing teachers and positive influences in public education and extracurricular activities. Ever since then, I have keenly observed graceful people and have been in awe of the human body and its movement capabilities. I learned at the age of eight to "breathe like a cat with my belly" when I sang and danced in the Andrew Lloyd Webber musical *Cats*. Those childhood experiences have informed how I watch people move and breathe.

I was fortunate to have had the opportunity to take a sports medicine class in high school, and fell in love with the field. I found a career that integrated science, competition, and compassion. I logged hundreds of hours watching athletes practice and play as an athletic training student. I was able to study how these elite and graceful athletes moved. (Not to mention all the years of watching Friday-night football games from the bandstand!) Being on the sidelines of sports is special. The relationship that develops between an athlete and the person taping their ankle is unique. I often knew when an athlete was hurt (and trying to hide it to stay on the field) before the coach did. At the age of 18, I knew I wanted to become a physical therapist. My teacher and mentor encouraged me to pursue this career and said, "If you get your undergraduate degree in athletic training and your graduate degree in physical therapy, you can write your own ticket." He was absolutely correct. I am aware of how uncommon my experience was.

I went on to earn my Bachelor of Science in Athletic Training/ Sports Medicine and scored a college job at the age of 23, as an assistant athletic trainer in the Midwest, while I applied to graduate school in physical therapy. I was accepted the next year to the masters program at an osteopathic school, which was also fortunate. The school's mission—humanism—and the emphasis on manual therapy shaped my ideals as a caregiving clinician. It was during physical therapy school that I earned a certification in strength and conditioning and, more importantly, discovered yoga.

My "yoga moment" came unexpectedly in graduate school while studying in Southern California at Western University of Health Sciences. As students, we were given gym memberships. Honestly, I was procrastinating from studying for the Strength and Conditioning Certification exam. I had finished my workout at the same time as a stretching class started. Of course I joined, as every aspiring physical therapist knows the value of a good cooldown! The class itself was not memorable; it was probably a basic hatha yoga class. However, during the final *savasana* (corpse pose)—the traditional resting pose in most lineages—I had an out-of-body experience. I felt my body lying on the cold gym floor on a thin beach towel, but in my mind's eye, I had floated to the ceiling and could see the entire gym floor and the basketball game next door. My consciousness expanded so greatly that I felt I was floating in the clouds above Mount Baldy.

The teacher eventually guided us back into our bodies. The lights came on and she bid us farewell. I was left wondering, "Did everyone experience that?" From that moment on, I have been a student of yoga and its philosophy. For years, I kept my secret yoga experience to myself. I was doing just fine in graduate school on the orthopedic track. Privately, however, yoga was my savior when times got tough.

Early in my physical therapy career, my sports medicine field experience was valued greatly by colleagues, and I enjoyed working in the outpatient orthopedic rehabilitation setting. However, I wasted a lot of time and energy attempting to justify the breathing techniques I offered patients to help cope with their surgical situations. Why? Because at that time, there was no room for nurturing language in a competitive sports clinic. In fact, it was considered a sign of weakness, and I was laughed at by my colleagues.

I went silent; yet I persisted. I also learned more skillful ways of teaching. The breathing techniques I shared were justified by science, but I couldn't use yogic or poetic language in front of my colleagues. So I became expert at translating yogic concepts into sports medicine language. Whatever I was doing to help clients labeled as "difficult" was working. Little did they know that yoga was the secret ingredient. While the sports medicine world was becoming more focused and one-pointed—like orthopedic surgeons specializing in a single body part—I was tasked with helping clients presenting with multiple injuries in their bodies simultaneously. I had to prioritize treatment plans and figure out where to start when treating people with a variety of persistent musculoskeletal injuries.

To do this, I used a global, holistic approach with my clients, simultaneously looking through the lenses of orthopedic physical therapy, athletic training, performance enhancement, yoga, and rehabilitation. I started centrally and cleared the spine first. Very often, patients who came in for a chronic lower extremity issue (anywhere in the leg) presented with a past or current lower back issue. In the early 2000s, the trend was to focus on strengthening the deep abdominal muscles in rehabilitation for back pain. This helped some people, but was not the magic resolution.

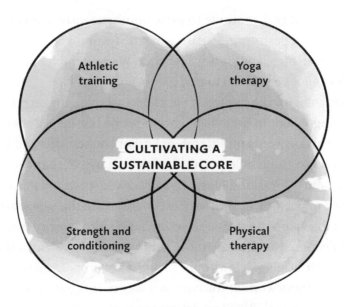

Athletic training

Yoga therapy

CULTIVATING A SUSTAINABLE CORE

Strength and conditioning

Physical therapy

CREATING A SUSTAINABLE CORE

The trunk and its supporting muscles work together in a sophisticated symphony, and the abdominal muscles do not work in solo. Decades of observing the different ways in which bodies coordinate their trunk stability led to my integrated view on the muscles of the core and to the ideas presented in this book. Clients who came in for an upper extremity issue (anywhere in the arm) often presented with less-than-optimal function in the neck or elsewhere on the spine. I became skilled at treating the spine and the extremities simultaneously. This approach came naturally when treating the client as a complete person with a whole body, as opposed to a bag of injured body parts with a brain. I explained in detail why I was doing a particular treatment, which empowered clients to participate in their own healing process. For many years, I have been riding the front wave of a paradigm shift already in motion. I taught patients to heal themselves. Rehabilitation is not a passive process; I help people learn how to listen to their own bodies in order to heal their physical ailments. I see myself simply as a guide or teacher. My professional offerings are integrative by nature. Legally, I cannot take off my physical therapy hat, as this is my highest professional level of responsibility. I continue to exist simultaneously as an athletic trainer and a performing artist at heart. I cannot separate these aspects from myself or the way I practice. We are complex organisms which cannot be reduced to parts.

Returning to the request from clients to share my secrets, just which ingredient in the rehabilitation recipe box helped them the most? The answer is multifaceted. I tailor the sessions and home programs to the whole person in front of me. Perhaps it's also because during sessions, I intentionally create space and make time to listen to people's stories. Maybe I could create this safe space for clients to explore their true selves because I also *practice* yoga and self-reflection. I am human, too. Clients sometimes ask for a simple formula for healing. I don't offer that. What I propose instead is an expanded framework of the core as a way to integrate the biopsychosocial-spiritual (BPSS) model with yoga, movement therapy, and physical rehabilitation.

Synchronicity led me to start my own practice. In 2006, California passed direct access laws for consumers to seek physical therapy directly for wellness. Since I already had earned and maintained multiple national certifications, I didn't have to do anything extra to show that I was qualified as a wellness practitioner. This was my opportunity to be independent from the traditional clinic model and open a private physical therapy office.

One thing I use in the studio to assess the client is palpation. To be clear, palpation is out of the scope of practice for most wellness practitioners. Massage therapists, physical therapists, occupational therapists, chiropractors, and other licensed health care providers who are trained in this should have clients sign a "consent to treat" form *and* obtain verbal permission to touch prior to touching clients, every time. As a patient, student, or client of yoga, you always have the right to refuse to be touched.

For years, I played percussion in the local symphony. As a percussionist, my sense of touch and vibration is highly refined, which informs my manual therapy skills. Fun fact: I stopped playing percussion for the local symphony in 2006 when I started my own side gig. As soon as this manuscript is complete, I will rejoin! While an important element of my practice, music therapy and palpation skills are beyond the scope of this book. My practice focuses on the intersection of physical therapy, athletic training, sports conditioning, manual therapy, and yoga. To simplify, I find myself teaching the same five concepts to everyone:

- **Bony core:** Alignment for centering
- **Muscular core:** Core muscle coordination
- **Breathing core:** Breath efficiency
- **Mindful core:** Movement awareness
- **Energetic core:** Subtle energy flow

How to Use This Book

This book is a window into how I assess my clients' needs using the BPSS model. It is evidence-based support for why I choose these reduced parts to examine the whole. If you find yourself getting bogged down by any of the research or technical discussion in Part II, please feel free to skim through to the end of each chapter. After discussing the bony core, muscular core, breathing core, mindful core, and energetic core concepts in Part II, I provide practical demonstrations and progressive instructions for experiencing the concepts within your own body in Part III. There, you will find more practical examples of the main concepts and exercises to explore.

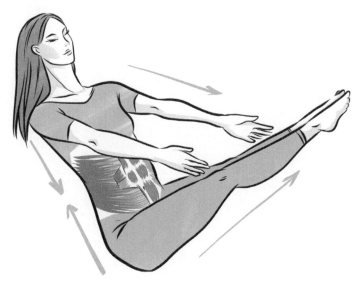

NAVASANA

Let's journey together, moving from awareness of bone to muscle, muscle to breath, breath to mindfulness, and mindfulness to subtle energy flow. From the tangible to the ethereal, and perhaps ultimately to Spirit or Universal Consciousness. Let's cultivate a sustainable core. Whether you are a movement therapist or simply someone who lives in a body, I hope you will find a helpful nugget that motivates a spark of change in your movement habits and breathing patterns which leads to greater balance between effort and ease.

Part I

CORE FOUNDATIONS

1

INTRODUCTION
TO THE CORE

I define the core of the body as the trunk, and the core *muscles* as all the muscles that attach to the trunk. In the literature, the core is not uniformly defined. It is stated that "numerous muscles make up the complex known as core muscles."[1] One study[2] names the "core muscles" to include only superficial muscles (the rectus abdominis, external oblique, and erector spinae muscles) because they are easy to study with electromyography (EMG) surface electrodes. The core is more often divided into two muscular units: the *outer core*, which includes large muscles that cross several joints, including the erector spinae, rectus abdominis, and external oblique muscles, and the *inner core* canister or cylinder composed of the pelvic floor, diaphragm, transverse abdominis, and multifidus muscles.

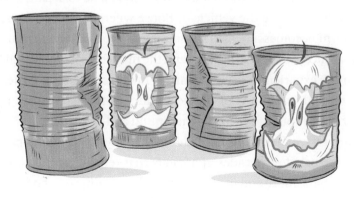

FIGURE 1.1 THE INNER CORE

I have a broader, deeper view of the core, dividing it into five lenses: bony core, muscular core, breathing core, mindful core, and energetic core. This view allows for discussion of specific aspects of the core, while recognizing that all five are always connected.

In Western or European academia and sciences (as opposed to the esoteric Eastern traditions), a technique or modality is tested in double-blind, dualistic, peer-reviewed studies to be valid. The standard is to reduce a complex phenomenon into discrete pieces to compare them and create reproducible and consistent results. One pain psychologist remarks: "Western medicine has incorrectly, and dangerously, divided humans into two disconnected entities: mind ('mental') and body ('physical')."[3] The human mind and body are not dualistic.

This book expands the view of the core, a perspective which has arisen from combining multiple disciplines. This perspective can be used as a framework to integrate the body, mind, and breath into musculoskeletal rehabilitation. The layers influence each other. Sometimes, small adjustments in one lens of focus can have a big impact on the larger picture.

In the same way that *asana*, or yoga postures, can be a gateway into the spiritual practice of yoga, physical therapy is an entry point of broader change for clients who come to an integrated private practice ostensibly to heal their material body, or "Earth Suit." Why do I call our physical-material body the Earth Suit? In the context of yoga, our body–mind–spirit are inseparable. If we were able to separate them, our body would be the vehicle or house where mind/spirit resides. The term becomes a light-hearted reference point when discussing pain science, theoretical physics, and the mysteries of life with clients.

In my experience, people come to my practice because they are dealing with some sort of physical injury or persistent pain issue. Their body is out of sync with their mind and spirit. Since graduate school, I have maintained a wider lens in my treatment approach. Over the past few decades, it appears that rehabilitation clinicians have become more and more specialized in treating one body part at a time. However, the incidence of multiple musculoskeletal injuries in athletes[4] and the general population remains prevalent and is manageable.[5, 6] Chronic low back pain (cLBP) is a leading cause of disability, and usual treatment is often ineffective. The incidence of low back and neck pain is on the rise and is a burden on the health care system.[7] The opioid crisis grew with this rise. In a white paper, the International Association of Yoga Therapists suggests that "The primary problem is misunderstood. Opioid misuse, addiction, overdose, and death are currently the main drivers of interventions, and these issues must be addressed; however, they are symptoms of larger systemic dysfunctions rather than the primary problem."[8] I agree that we have a pain crisis, versus an opioid problem. Non-pharmacological interventions such as physical therapy,[9] and complementary and alternative interventions such as yoga and mindfulness-based-stress reduction (MBSR), are now included in pain-management best practices by the United States Department of Health and Human Services.[10]

Integrated and Holistic Rehabilitation Trends
Regional Interdependence Model
To address the cLBP prevalence, specialization of clinicians, and the pain crisis (and lifestyle-choice diseases which are preventable) there is a new evidence-based model for rehabilitation specialists to consider, called regional interdependence.[11]

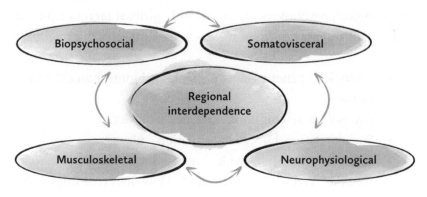

FIGURE I.2 REGIONAL INTERDEPENDENCE

Regional interdependence is "a clinical model of musculoskeletal assessment and intervention. The underlying premise of this model is that seemingly unrelated impairments in remote anatomical regions of the body may contribute to and be associated with a patient's primary report of symptoms."[12] It recognizes that the different systems in the body, such as the somatovisceral, neurophysiological, and musculoskeletal systems, are interrelated and cannot be separated from each other. This model allows us to expand our clinical view and is in line with a holistic approach. The regional interdependence model includes the biopsychosocial-spiritual (BPSS) model.

Biopsychosocial-Spiritual Model

We cannot make changes in one realm without the entire organism responding and adapting. "Healthcare changes have required PTs [physical therapists] to adapt to a biopsychosocial-spiritual model (BPSS) for improved patient outcomes."[13] This model recognizes that one aspect of our being influences another.[14, 15, 16, 17, 18, 19, 20, 21] It is now acknowledged that "An integrative, comprehensive bio-psy-cho-social-spiritual (BPSS) framework is needed for reexamining, preventing, and addressing the root causes of chronic/persistent pain and suffering…" This includes "recognizing…outcomes such as quality of life, flourishing, and well-being."[22]

In a foundational free-access yoga therapy course for health professionals, Matthew Taylor defines the biopsychosocial-spiritual model as "A theoretical framework that assumes a complex concert of biological, psychological, social, and spiritual factors from an individual's unique health status."[23] Some examples of this might be:

- Biological: genetics, age, physiology, biomechanical/linear causality
- Psychological: emotions, attitudes, behaviors
- Social: relationships, living situation, culture
- Spiritual: how an individual makes sense of their life situation (i.e.: Who/What/Why am I? How does that inform my actions?).

Pain is complex, and the historical biomedical understanding of pain inaccurately reduces and endorses a linear relationship between noxious stimuli and pain. A study by Stilwell and Harman put it this way: "From a Cartesian dualist perspective, pain occurs in an immaterial mind. From a reductionist perspective, pain is often considered to be 'in the brain.'"[24] The BPSS model attempts to address this, and while this model is useful, we don't want to use it in a reductionist way. "There is a lack of research conceptualising how physiotherapy applies the bio-psycho-social model in research and practice."[25] An "enactive" approach has been suggested, where "pain is a relational and emergent process of sense-making through a lived body that is inseparable from the world that we shape and that shapes us."[26]

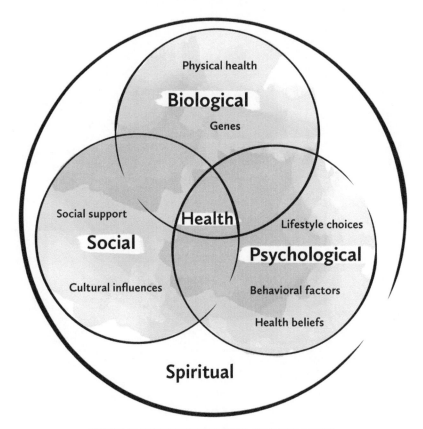

FIGURE 1.3 THE BIOPSYCHOSOCIAL-SPIRITUAL MODEL

Health care providers don't have to reinvent the wheel when addressing the complexity of chronic pain. Yoga is inherently non-dualistic and yoga therapy already incorporates the BPSS model. Wims et al. (2017) note that "Therapeutic yoga may provide an opportunity for PTs [physical therapists] to expand their role in health and wellness and chronic disease management."[27] In the white paper by the International Association of Yoga Therapists, they affirm "that yoga therapy is an essential component of the multidisciplinary undertaking that will be required to improve patient outcomes and alter the trajectory of the public health crisis of poorly addressed pain."[28]

2

INTRODUCTION TO YOGA

There are many definitions of yoga. In Sanskrit, the word "yoga" itself comes from *yog*, which literally translates to "yoke" or "combine." One of my favorite explanations of the aim of yoga is to attain a mental state free from disturbance. We do that by working with the breath as we bend and twist and stretch the physical body to help train the mind. Yoga includes the physical body as one of the many layers to consider, or ways to access one's center and gain spiritual enlightenment. Ironically, though the definition of yoga is "to yoke or join," the actual goal of yoga is to separate and dissolve *prakriti* (matter) and to merge into the *atman* (the higher self) or *purusa* (spirit). According to Patanjali's Yoga Sutra 2.46, *sthira-sukham asanam*, that is, yoga *asana*, or postures, should be stable and comfortable, or seeking the balance between "effort" and "ease."[1] Yoga is liberation of the soul; it is a spiral and full circle. Again, it is not simple or dualistic.

It is well documented that yoga can help a variety of conditions;[2] for example:

- depression, anxiety, stress[3, 4, 5]
- hypertension, heart disease, asthma, diabetes[6]
- breast cancer and inflammation in cancer survivors[7]
- pregnancy, prenatal and postpartum depression[8]
- pain syndromes, including arthritis, headaches, and low back pain[9]
- multiple sclerosis, human immunodeficiency virus (HIV) symptoms[10]

- post-traumatic stress disorder (PTSD), balance, obesity, osteo-porosis, Parkinson's.[11]

Yoga "appears to be as safe or safer when compared to other exercise types" based on the overall injury rate per 1000 practice hours,[12] yet many rehabilitation professionals are hesitant to prescribe yoga as an intervention. However, in meta-analyses, researchers found yoga to be more effective than control conditions. Yoga as a treatment intervention was found to be so much more effective than the other exercise types that researchers concluded, "Having established the physical and mental health benefits of yoga makes it ethically questionable to assign participants to inactive control groups."[13] In other words, they found it unethical not to include yoga in the control group to compare treatment interventions.

What is it about yoga that is so special? "Yoga considers that every individual is not merely limited to only the physical level of existence but is made up of a multi-fold universal nature."[14] In yoga, concepts like *pancha kosha* (the fivefold aspect of our existence) and *trisharira* (the threefold aspect of our bodily nature) help us understand that we are more than our physical bodies. Our multidimensional natures result from a dynamic interaction of all the layers.[15] We cannot separate our body from the environment. We cannot separate our cells and the working physiology from our body. We are made of interconnected, complex layers.

Koshas

In the Indian spiritual-philosophical *pancha maya kosha* model, the human body has inseparable energetic layers which surround our soul. These five layers, or sheaths, called *koshas*, can be thought of as our five bodies or "coverings" of the self/*atman*.[16] The pure light of our spiritual soul essence can be described as being covered or enveloped by five sheaths. We can think of these layers as parts of our bodies that assimilate the food we eat, our breath, the thoughts we think, how we discern those thoughts, and then how we connect to the whole.

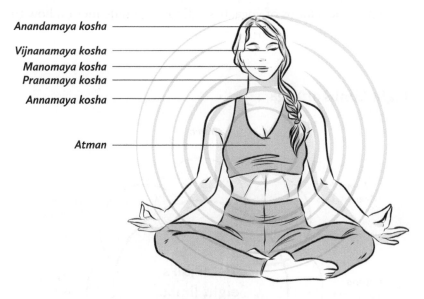

Anandamaya kosha
Vijnanamaya kosha
Manomaya kosha
Pranamaya kosha
Annamaya kosha

Atman

FIGURE 2.I THE *KOSHAS*

Roughly, the layers that cover the self/*atman* can be translated to:

- **Physical:** Material body (common entry point to yoga in modern times). Food/Earth element. *Annamaya kosha.*
- **Energetic:** *Pranic* body (energy from metabolized food and oxygen). Vital sheath/Water element. *Pranamaya kosha.*
- **Emotional:** Mental-social-emotional-body (our daily mind). Mental sheath/Fire element. *Manomaya kosha.*
- **Intellectual:** Wisdom discrimination body (higher mind; the witness consciousness). Intellect/intuitive sheath/Air element. *Vijnanamaya kosha.*
- **Spiritual:** Bliss Body (being with nature, connection with the Divine Soul, enlightenment). Ether/Space element. *Anandamaya kosha.*

Again, these layers are inseparable and each layer informs the other. Yoga is a path to spiritual bliss. In Patanjali's *Yoga Sutra*, the eightfold path toward liberation is called *ashtanga*, which literally means "eight limbs" (*ashta* = eight, *anga* = limb). "These eight steps, commonly known as the 8 limbs of yoga, basically act as guidelines on how to live a meaningful and purposeful life."[17]

Eight Limbs of Yoga

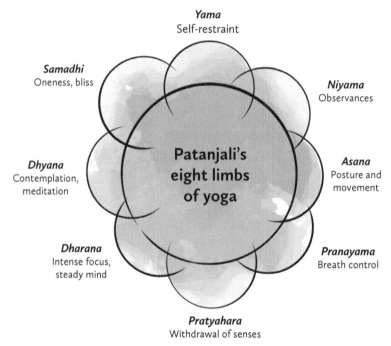

FIGURE 2.2 PATANJALI'S EIGHT LIMBS OF YOGA

By practicing these eight limbs, we may temporarily experience one-ness (*samadhi*, or bliss), but we still have to move, breathe, think, and interact with our surroundings in our daily lives. Yoga considers how we behave within ourselves and how we behave within our community and our society (the *yamas* and *niyamas*). It is a practice, and it is not linear. Again, the layers are inseparable. When people think about yoga, images of people in awkward poses, or *asana* (the third limb), might be visualized. Note that *asana* actually refers to "the posture that brings comfort and steadiness. Any pose that brings this comfort and steadiness is an *asana*."[18] The aim of yoga is not to produce the twisted pretzel images one might imagine.

To make those awkward poses seem easy, the practitioner probably also practiced a steady mind and breath. Yet, as I have suggested,
yoga and the path to freedom from suffering are a nonlinear journey.
I think of the journey as a spiral. We meditate, we challenge our
bodies and minds physically, and we strive to be good citizens to
ourselves and communities. Just when we accomplish a goal, we
often find ourselves back on the mat or meditation cushion again
learning how to be human. Just as *asana* is often an entry point to
the practice of yoga, an expanded look at the core can be a gateway
to understanding rehabilitation of the whole body.

3

THE CORE: BASIC PRINCIPLES AND TERMINOLOGY

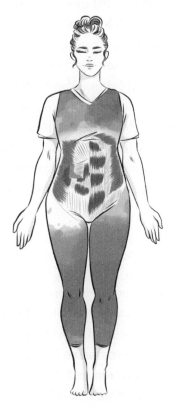

FIGURE 3.1 THE ABDOMINAL MUSCLES

The term "core" conjures up many different images. During my undergraduate kinesiology studies, we thought of the core as the trunk muscles. This is true, yet the core is more refined than that. The term "has been used to refer to the trunk, or more specifically the lumbo-pelvic region of the body."[1] It is also "defined as the axial skeleton and all soft tissues with a proximal attachment on the axial skeleton."[2] The axial skeleton, by definition, includes the bones in the skull, spine, and rib cage. I include the pelvis as part of the trunk.

Layers of the Core

Core muscles with attachments to the lumbo-sacral region of the trunk include the lumbar multifidus, erector spinae, quadratus lumborum, external oblique abdominis, internal oblique abdominis, rectus abdominis, transverse abdominis, psoas major, pelvic floor muscles, and diaphragm. I define the *core region* of the body as the "trunk" (pelvis, abdomen, and thorax) and I define the *core muscles* as "all the muscles which attach to the trunk." A basic understanding of anatomy is assumed for this book, but please don't let the names of muscles steer you away from the concepts. While the primary audience of this book is movement professionals, I hope also to lay out basic principles anyone could use when learning to move their body more efficiently.

Planes of Movement

When discussing the relative positions or relationships between body parts, kinesiologists use standard terminology for the planes and axes of movement in space.[3] Imagine that you are standing with good posture, arms at your side, palms facing forward. This is *anatomical position*. It's not a natural position, but it is the starting point from which we define movement. Note that it is also *tadasana*, or mountain pose, in yoga. Now, let's place three imaginary planes of glass through our body along the three axes in space.

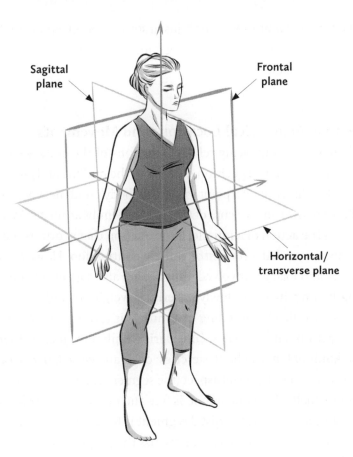

FIGURE 3.2 PLANES OF THE BODY

The plane that divides our body into front and back halves is called the *frontal plane*. If we were to side-bend our trunk to the left or right, we would be moving in the frontal plane (around a transverse axis).

The sheet that separates our body into equal left and right halves is the *sagittal plane*. When we flex our spine forward or extend it in a backbend, we are moving in the sagittal plane (about a horizontal axis).

When we twist or rotate our head and trunk, we are moving in the *horizontal plane* (also known as the transverse plane) around a vertical axis. The names of the planes remain the same when we deviate from anatomical position, but the forces of gravity change on the body. In real life, we move through all planes of motion, also called *tri-planar* motion. This is just a starting point, and we will take advantage of these facts when we get into more specific interventions later in the book.

Relative Anatomical Locations and Movements

When we are comparing relative locations of the body, we use the word *distal* to note a position *away* from the midline and *proximal* to name the direction of a point *toward* the body's midline. For example, relative to the trunk or core of the body, the limbs are distal. When we discuss the action of a muscle, a contraction that shortens the muscle fibers is called a *concentric* muscle contraction. However, when gravity and load get involved, muscles are also capable of controlled lengthening (imagine slowly lowering a weight toward the ground). This controlled lengthening of a muscle is termed *eccentric* muscle contraction. Finally, when considering limb movements, there are two kinds of kinetic chain exercises: open and closed. In *open kinetic chain* exercises, the distal aspect (the segment furthest away from the body), usually the hand or foot, is free and not fixed to an object. In a *closed-chain exercise*, the distal segment is fixed, or stationary. These terms come in handy when we discuss the progression of exercise.

All of the clients I work with want to move with more ease. Some call themselves patients and have persistent pain. Others are athletes or people who practice yoga and have a physical goal or perceived limitation. Many have recovered from ligament or soft tissue injuries, both acute and chronic. Protecting their ligaments from end-range injury and prolonged load seems to be a recurring theme. They all have the common goal of being more resilient and adaptable to movement in their material body. Just like a client might go to a psychotherapist to learn and practice new thought patterns, clients might come to holistic and integrated physical therapy (PT) to learn novel movement patterns.

The bodies of people who come to the studio for help have adapted to a protective movement pattern. Initially, this movement pattern (such as limping) can get someone through their day. However, once a tissue injury is healed, if they still expect pain, the limp can persist and become habitual.[4] When a client shows up in my studio, they have already informed me of their goals and their limiting beliefs about these goals. Their goals are often movement oriented. I provide a safe setting for them to be heard and to re-explore movement. For example, in the initial paperwork, I ask:

- What services attracted you to Body Temple? (check all that apply):
  - ❏ Traditional Physical Therapy Evaluation and Treatment
  - ❏ Manual Body Work including joint and tissue mobilization ("PT Massage")
  - ❏ Personal Training/Strength and Conditioning and Athletic Training
  - ❏ Yoga and Pilates.

Their answers help me meet them where they are, and inform me what language and vocabulary might best resonate with the person in front of me. The answers can be very telling. For instance, they might strike through "Yoga and Pilates" darkly, as if their pen were scratching out the existence of alternative lenses altogether. I tend to start with solid science and medical terminology with this group. Other people only check the yoga therapy box. The ones who check *all* the boxes tend to be the most open-minded. However, I do not want to make any causal assumptions. No matter what boxes they check, I inquire about their needs. Sometimes people just need to be heard before they allow themselves to make changes and shift their perspectives. Just as pain is complex and unique to an individual, the journey of rehabilitation is also complex and unique to an individual.

The common principles I teach are applicable on many levels. The idea is to get the client to move freely again; I offer a physical launching point. While one can enter from any lens, I try to let the client lead the path of a session, and meet them at the level of awareness they come in with. We set goals together. Clients seek advice on how to move therapeutically, for *physical* therapy. I often use yoga as a modality. Yoga offers a lens for movement assessment and can be turned into therapy or homework to practice a new way of moving or breathing. It can be used to illuminate habitual patterns and apply this awareness and turn it into self-healing medicine. In therapy sessions, I observe clients' movements and *simultaneously* apply these five lenses:

- Are they protecting/controlling their ligaments at end-ranges of motion?
- Are they managing their abdominal pressures effectively?
- Are they breathing while they move?
- Are their chosen movements thoughtful?
- Are they open-minded to the mysteries of the Universe and the possibility of subtle energy flow?

In other words, I consistently observe their bony alignment, core muscle coordination, breathing efficiency, mindfulness, and open-mindedness with their movements. If there is a glitch in one of these cogs in the wheel, then the whole machine is inefficient. Information gained from these observations gives me insight into the interventions I might use.

My experiences and observations have led me to a helpful framework of conceptualizing the core as five separate parts, which link into the elements of Earth, Water, Fire, Air, and the invisible life energy, *prana*, using both an anatomical/kinesiological/biomechanical and a yogic lens. For that reason, the chapters in Part II of the book are organized into the five components:

- bony/passive tissue (passive structure) (Chapter 4)
- muscle/active tissue (dynamic tissue) (Chapter 5)
- breathing parts (breath mechanics) (Chapter 6)
- mindful components (neurological physiology) (Chapter 7)
- energetic-spiritual parts (the invisible life energy) (Chapter 8).

From the more tangible bones and structural body to the mind and more subtle or energetic body, all the elements work together to make up the whole, just like the inseparable layers of the trunk make the core.

This may be a challenging paradigm for some traditionally trained physical therapists and medical doctors. On the other hand, as a kinesiologist, some may see me as too rigid or reductionist. My hope is to find the middle ground. At the very least, may these words plant a seed and provide an alternate glimpse of how the BPSS model might work. Perhaps some of the magic I have witnessed and experienced professionally and personally can be used as a tool for you to find a comfortable seat in your own core.

Since the core is a section of our material body, we could apply the concept of layers or sheaths to the core. Let's divide the ingredients of the core into different yogic elements:

- bony core: Earth and Water (*kapha*)
- muscular core: Fire and Water (*pitta*)
- breathing core: Air and Ether (*vata*)
- mindful core: Ether and Space (*vata*).
- energetic core: Energy (*prana*).

According to Ayurvedic medicine, the world is comprised of five elements—ether/space, water, earth, fire, and air. A combination of each element results in three bodily humors, or *doshas*—*vata*, *kapha*, and *pitta*—which we each possess in combination, with one being dominant. These *doshas* determine our Ayurvedic constitution.

Vata is mainly air and space, and those with a dominant *vata dosha* are usually slim, energetic, and creative. *Kapha* is earth- and water-based. People with this dominant *dosha* are typically strong, thick-boned, caring, slower-moving individuals. The *pitta dosha* is based on fire and water. People with *pitta* dominance are said to be athletic, fiery, and competitive. Our *dosha* make-up defines our needs for optimal physiological, mental, and emotional health, and can be useful in making appropriate diet, exercise, and lifestyle choices.

No matter how we divide it, tri-doshic (three layers) or five-fold, we are made of inseparable material and energetic-spiritual parts. We are made up of a spectrum of matter from the material to the intangible, energetic mysteries. In seeking health, we strive for balance and harmony between all the layers.

Part II

THE SUSTAINABLE CORE

4

THE BONY CORE

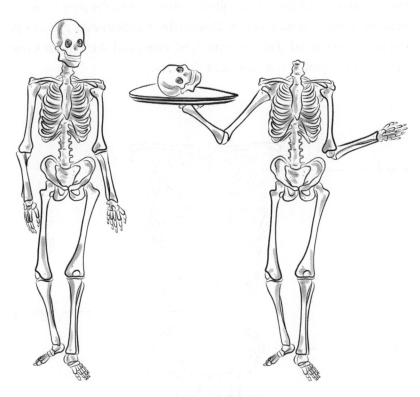

FIGURE 4.1 THE SKELETON

Bony Core Anatomy

When we divide the expanded view of the core into five yogic elements from tangible to ethereal, the first section is composed of bones and *passive* soft tissue. I call this the bony core. Passive soft tissue is cartilage (the tissue that cushions and lines the bones where they articulate or touch other bones), ligaments, (which attach bone to bone), tendons (which attach muscle to bone), and fascia (the soft-tissue "wrapping" around organs, vessels, and muscles). One way to define the relevant bony core anatomy is through the following thought exercise:

First, let's look at our skeleton, remembering that it's three-dimensional. Imagine cutting off our heads like a Halloween character. Then, imagine that we cut off the arms and legs. What's left is a three-dimensional bony core cylinder made up of the pelvis, vertebrae, ribs, and scapulae bones. Essentially, the *bony core cylinder* is the traditional axial skeleton (spine, rib cage, and skull) minus the skull plus the pelvis, scapulae, and clavicles.

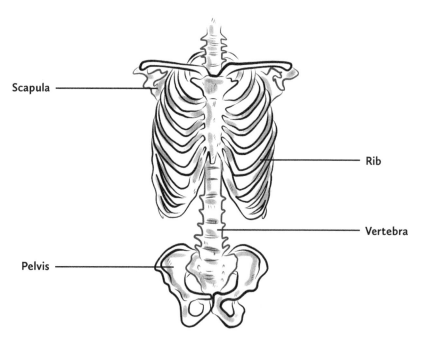

Scapula

Rib

Vertebra

Pelvis

FIGURE 4.2 THE BONY CORE CYLINDER

This bony core is a three-dimensional canister, or cylinder, like a tin can.

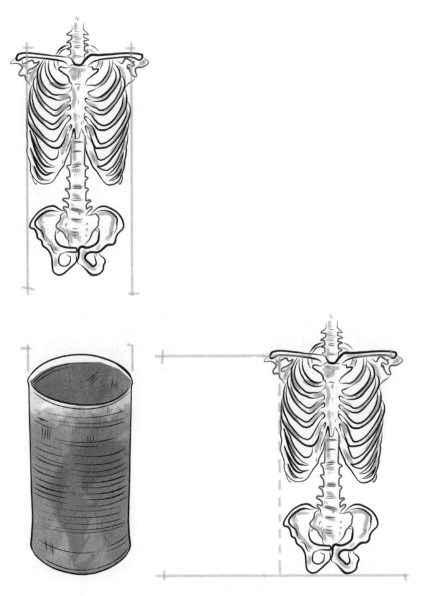

FIGURE 4.3 THE CORE CYLINDER

The bottom of the can is represented in the body by the pelvic bones. The bones of the vertebrae stack up and make a vertical pole or "stick." The 24 ribs radiate out from each side of the 12 thoracic vertebrae in the mid-section of the "pole." In other words, the axial skeleton plus the scapulae, clavicles, and pelvis make up the bony core. The scapulae, or shoulder blades, rest on the rib cage. Think of anatomy as a map of our physical body. The bones are the foundation of the musculoskeletal system, just like the foundation of a house. The bony core is the scaffolding of the sustainable core, and its *alignment* affects the relationship of the team of muscles that attach to it. If our bony core is not aligned in a centered manner, the soft tissue anchored to it is unbalanced. We can compare this to a dented can. If there is a dent in the bony core cylinder, the muscles attached to the foundation have different length–tension relationships from one side of the can to the other. The alignment of the bony core matters.

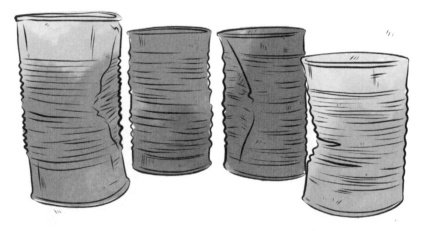

FIGURE 4.4 MISALIGNMENT

To illustrate, I invite you to imagine someone with scoliosis (excessive lateral curvature in the spine) or hyperkyphosis (extreme hunching in the thoracic spine). You can see that *if the bony core is off-center, the entire core system potential is altered.*

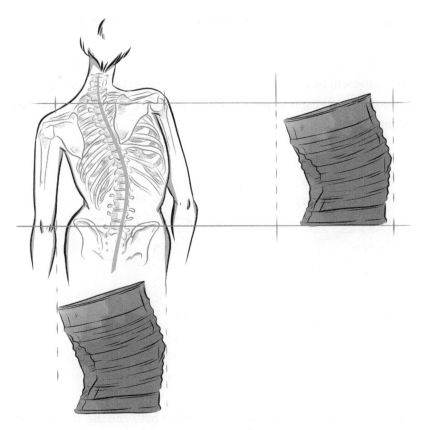

FIGURE 4.5 SCOLIOSIS

Note how the rotation and curve of the spine affects the alignment of the rib cage. This in turn alters the symmetry of the bony core, as well as the position of the anchor points of the core muscles. We will unpack the muscular and functional implications and anatomical detail further in Chapter 5, The Muscular Core. For now, let's continue to focus on the concept of the scaffolding of a cylinder-shaped building as our body's bony core analogy.

The longevity of a suspension bridge over a windy canyon depends on smooth interfacing surfaces, just as the joints of the human body must respond to wear and tear. If the end of a beam has a jagged surface where it articulates (or touches) the metal next to it, the shear and compression forces will wear unevenly. The human body is resilient and usually adapts to the increased load by building more bone or soft tissue. This in itself does not lead to pain or decreased performance. However, if the integrity of a bone is weak, such as in osteoporosis, or the connective tissue is frail for various reasons, the tissue will be compromised. A compression fracture or ruptured tendon might result when the forces are too high for the tissue to maintain integrity.

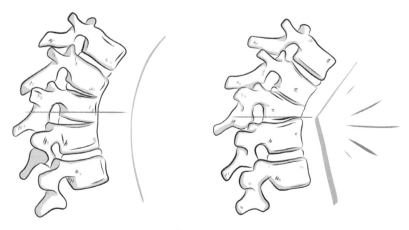

FIGURE 4.6 SQUISHED VERTEBRA

Every joint has a position in which contact between the articulating structures is minimal. This is called the *open-packed position* of a joint. In manual therapy, this is the optimal position to assess joint integrity because it is the position where the soft tissue is on slack. The opposite, the *closed-packed position* of a joint, is the position in which there is maximum congruency (or maximum available surface contact) of the articular surfaces and joint stability is derived from the alignment of the bones. When considering the bony core as a single collective joint, the concept of *neutral spine* best approximates the open-pack position of the core. I recommend using this position as a starting point or physical entry point to movement awareness.

In sports training and performance enhancement, we train the body to withstand high forces of impact by *gradually* building up muscle strength and resilience in all *planes* of motion and through all *ranges* of motion, including the *end*-ranges. Elite athletes don't become strong, skilled, and resilient overnight; they have to start somewhere. For those just beginning on their movement journey, or those using movement as rehabilitation, I don't recommend starting with high loads at extreme end-ranges of motion. When learning new movement patterns, I recommend learning a centered posture as a calibration point. This centered *spinal* posture has historically been termed "neutral spine."

Neutral Spine

The spine is three-dimensional. Our physical body is like an onion; it has many functional layers. Let's peel that open. In physical therapy school, we were all loaned a "bone box" to take home and study during the term. It contained all the vertebrae, a skull, one leg, and one arm. My roommate and I spread the vertebrae out on our living room carpet and began to assemble our half skeletons like eager children dumping out pieces of a new puzzle. The thing that impressed me then, and stays with me to this day, is that no two vertebrae were the same size. There is only one correct way to put the vertebrae back together. And when they are reassembled correctly, beautiful curves emerge. Front and back views of the spine yield a vertical alignment, while side views reveal curves and a shock-absorbing spring in the neutral spine. Figure 4.7, from left to right, shows the back view, side view, and front view respectively.

We are not born with these curves. As infants, we exist in the fetal, spinal flexion position. In medical terminology, we say that we are born with a primary C-shaped curve in the spine. This primary curve is our kyphotic curve. As we develop and move our muscles against gravity, new curves develop in the spine. Lordotic curves emerge in our neck and low back as we learn to lift our heads, crawl, stand, and walk upright vertically against gravity.[1]

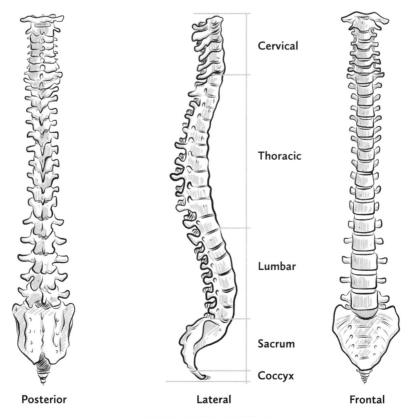

Posterior   Lateral   Frontal

FIGURE 4.7 SPINE ANATOMY

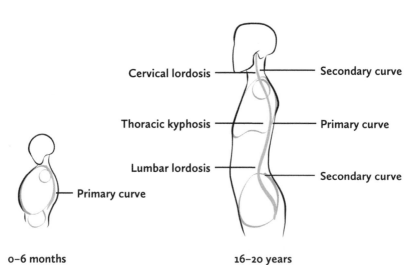

FIGURE 4.8 PRIMARY CURVES

The adult spine can respond to gravity's forces pulling down and balance them with ground reaction forces pushing up like a spring. The more length the spring/spine has, the more potential space there is to absorb the shocks and forces our spine encounters in daily life. This optimal adult spinal alignment is in the neutral spine zone.

Neutral spine is not absolute. It is a range, or neutral zone, or "a region of intervertebral motion around the neutral posture where little resistance is offered by the passive spinal column."[2] Just like in manual therapy, in yoga we begin by positioning a joint in its open packed position. I will often have clients begin a movement session by feeling their body in this neutral zone position.

Posture Discussion

The position of the ankle, pelvis, spine, rib cage, and skull affect core muscle recruitment.[3, 4, 5, 6] Spinal position affects lumbar loads and intervertebral disc pressure,[7, 8, 9, 10] posture affects breathing,[11] and lumbo-pelvic upright sitting posture with deep breathing affects core muscle recruitment.[12] Additionally, excessive thoracic kyphosis and misaligned head and trunk position makes intra-abdominal pressure (IAP) more difficult to manage correctly.[13, 14, 15, 16, 17, 18, 19] These combined factors can result in pelvic organ prolapse.[20] Clinically, I also see mismanagement of IAP commonly with hernias, intervertebral disc issues, and spinal joint (facet) arthritis.

Early in my career, I learned that "lumbo-pelvic neutral postures may have a positive influence on spinal stability... Therefore, posture may be important for rehabilitation in patients with LBP."[21] Furthermore, alteration of head and neck positions can have an immediate negative impact on respiratory function.[22] Research underscored this relationship. "Unlike obesity and physical activity, disorders of continence and respiration were strongly related to frequent back pain. This relationship may be explained by physiological limitations of co-ordination of postural, respiratory and continence functions of trunk muscles."[23] Another study suggested that it was important to "include the evaluation and treatment of faulty respiration in the

rehabilitation of chronic musculo-skeletal conditions, most notably cervical pain."[24] Breathing mechanics are influenced directly by
"Bio-mechanical factors such as rib head fixations or classical upper/
lower crossed patterns of muscle imbalance...[and] Psychosocial
factors such as chronic anxiety, anger or depression."[25]

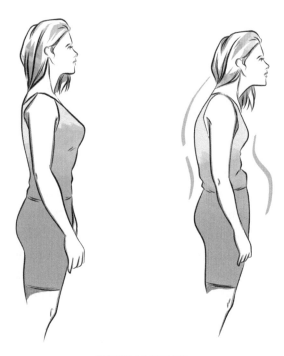

FIGURE 4.9 SLOUCH

I learned that a sedentary lifestyle plus faulty posture was correlated
with the weakening of core muscles, "which contributes to increased
incidence of musculoskeletal disorders (MSDs)."[26] One research study
even postulated that simply becoming *aware* of one own's posture
helped participants decrease their neck pain.[27] I clearly remember
one of my professors saying that just like "location, location, location"
is important in real estate, "posture, posture, posture" is important
in orthopedics. I leaned into this theory and have taught postural
alignment as part of movement therapy my entire career. In a recent
interview, physical therapist Susan Clinton said, "Postural alignment
does matter for performance—whatever that performance may be,"

but that the posture depends on the task and demands for breathing at hand.[28]

However, currently in the literature there is no causal evidence for perfect posture helping with low back pain.[29, 30] And lumbo-pelvic posture does not appear to have a significant effect on the timing of pelvic floor muscle (PFM) activation during coughing or load-catching tasks.[31] Having said that, "there is a wide range of good-quality literature to support the complex and biopsychosocial nature of chronic low-back pain beyond 'neutral' posture. Relying on a bio-medical paradigm to explain a complex biopsychosocial problem is inadequate."[32]

We are dynamic, moving, breathing creatures. So why am I dedicating an entire chapter to alignment? Biomechanics and posture *are* important when it comes to extreme, end-range positions under highly loaded conditions.[33] Traumatic fractures, and ligament and tendon ruptures, happen at extreme end-ranges of motion when the force is too high for the tissue to hold. There is an obvious mechanism of injury, such as the case in a knee ligament rupture when the angle of the knee supersedes its physical limits. If we land from a jump with our knee in an extremely twisted position (excessive valgus force) and the load and angle are too much for our muscles and tendons to absorb, the ligaments, which hold bones together, can't withstand the force, and rupture. This excessive valgus force when landing from a jump scenario is the classic mechanism of injury for an anterior cruciate ligament (ACL) sprain, which can take an injured athlete out of their sport to rehabilitate for several months.

Alignment of the knee may not be so important with low-load activities like distance running. For example, we see plenty of marathon runners with excessive foot pronation and valgus knee postures who have no complaints of pain. However, if this compensation originally derived from an attempt to avoid pain, one way out might be to practice an alignment that activates underused muscles, especially once the tissue has healed and this pattern has become habitual.

I still look at posture and alignment as a part of a movement analysis. So does physical therapist Shirley Sahrmann. "Though I am fully aware of the lack of evidence, I cannot imagine treating any patient without assessing posture or, more precisely, alignment," she noted.[34] Sahrmann discusses how we might be asking the wrong questions in regard to the relationship between pain and mechanics, and suggests that "Assessment of alignment impairments has to be an important step in designing an appropriate treatment program for correcting mechanical impairments."[35] However, the human body is multifaceted and complex, as are pain and performance improvements.

These two ideas can co-exist: first, there is an optimal midrange position for a task, and, second, there is individual postural variation in people. For example, there are many high-performing athletes who have three limbs or severe scoliosis (implying that they are not consistently moving through their neutral spine zone) without complaints of pain. Alignment is a common starting point for calibration, or self-assessment. *Alignment is individual and dynamic, and "posture" depends on the task at hand.*

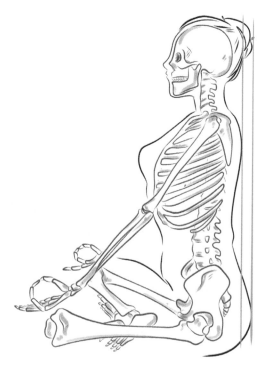

FIGURE 4.10 SEATED CROSS-LEGGED

How to Find a Neutral Spine Zone

One way to find neutral spine is to begin with neutral *pelvis*, because the position of the pelvis affects the position of the thoracic and lumbar curves.[36, 37] I often instruct clients to find a seated neutral pelvis and spine in this manner:

Sit at the edge of a chair with your feet firmly resting on the ground. Place your hands on the front of your pelvis. Use your fingertips to touch the pubic symphysis (PS) and the heels of your hands on the anterior superior iliac spine (ASIS) points [see Figure 4.11]. If there is too much flesh to feel those bony points, simply place your hands on top of the crests of the pelvis (the iliac crests) to get a sense of where the pelvis bones are.

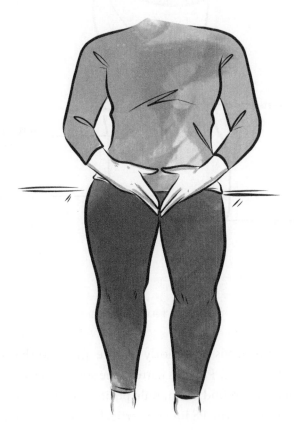

FIGURE 4.11 SEATED POSTURE

Either way, become aware of your "sitting bones" (ischial tuberosities) by finding these bones with your hands through your flesh. Then note these points contacting the chair's surface. Gently perform an anterior pelvic tilt [Figure 4.13A] by rocking the pelvis forward to arch your low back. This brings the "hip points" or ASIS of the pelvis in front of the pubic symphysis and yields an excessive lumbar arch.

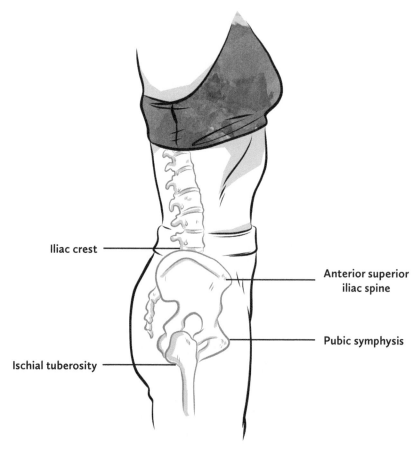

Iliac crest

Anterior superior
iliac spine

Pubic symphysis

Ischial tuberosity

FIGURE 4.12 PELVIS ALIGNMENT

Then tuck your pelvis posteriorly [Figure 4.13C] so that the ASIS points land behind the PS. This flattens the spine and eliminates any lumbar curve. Then find the middle position [Figure 4.13B], where the ASIS points and the PS line up vertically. This is neutral pelvis.

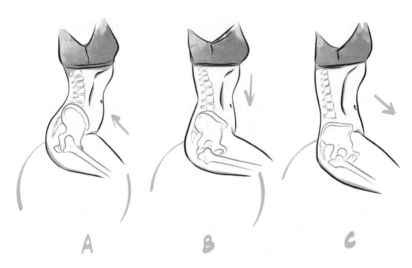

FIGURE 4.13 NEUTRAL PELVIS

Note that when the pelvis is in this middle position, a natural neutral lumbar curve emerges in the spine. Now, stack your rib cage and head vertically on top of your neutral pelvis, like a snow-person. Once you do this, the entire spine is in a neutral position and your three-dimensional bony core cylinder is also in neutral alignment.

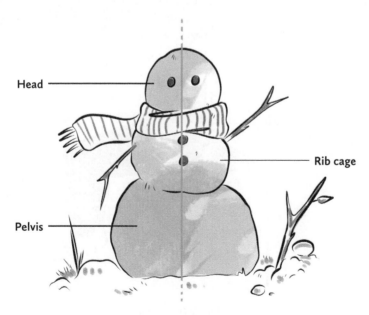

FIGURE 4.14 SNOW-PERSON

Another way we can find a neutral spine zone is by using a broomstick or dowel as an alignment guide. In strength training, we use movement screens as a functional evaluation standard in the functional movement system.[38, 39] One test used in this system to screen for hip and leg mobility is the "in-line lunge," where the dowel is placed behind the back touching the head, thoracic spine, and middle of the buttocks. I have adapted it for more general posture and function screening. I recommend holding the dowel in your palm and placing the back of the hand in the "small of the back," or the knuckles at the peak of the lumbar curve. Allow the pole to contact three different bony landmarks: the sacrum, the eighth thoracic vertebra (roughly the "bra-line"), and the skull.

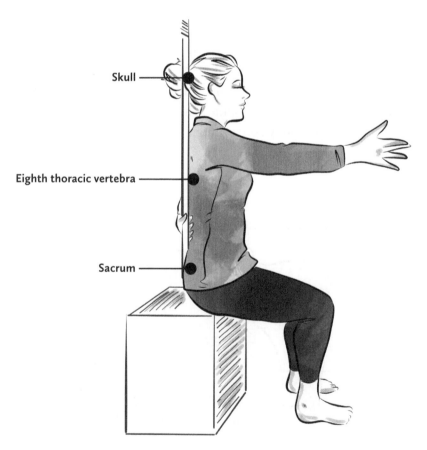

Skull

Eighth thoracic vertebra

Sacrum

FIGURE 4.15 SEATED POSTURE WITH DOWEL

Note that when we line up the body in this fashion, the neutral lumbar and cervical curves emerge. We can use this method to find good alignment in standing, too: see Figure 4.16.

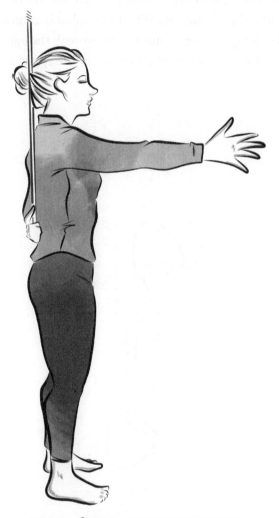

FIGURE 4.16 STANDING POSTURE WITH DOWEL

When we are standing, in neutral spine with our palms forward, we are in mountain pose or *tadasana*, which is a great gateway or centered entry position for many standing activities. If you don't have a broomstick or dowel handy, try standing with your back against a doorframe or wall corner, for self-assessment. The snow-person and broomstick alignments are just two of my favorite demonstrations to help clients experience a new center and posture calibration point. Another demonstration is to imagine that our thorax and pelvis are two parts of a plastic egg. When our spine is extended beyond neutral, this imaginary egg cannot close or seal; the egg is "open" in the front and a hinge force might collect in the spine or back body.

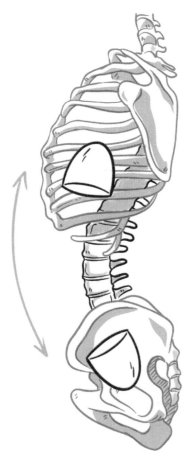

FIGURE 4.17 OPEN EGG

However, if we align our rib cage and pelvis so that the two halves of the imaginary egg align ("closed egg"), the spine aligns in a more neutral shape and, as we will learn in Chapter 5, The Muscular Core, the diaphragm muscles of the pelvis and thorax are positioned for better muscle length–tension relationship.

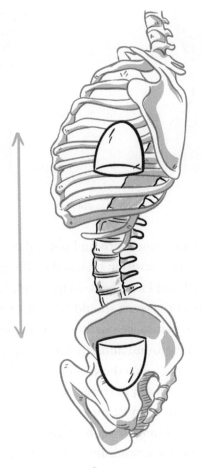

FIGURE 4.18 CLOSED EGG

When the egg shell is "open" in the front (anteriorly) this is also known as a "rib flare." I cue clients to "close the egg" (vertically) or "knit the lower ribs" (transversely) together in front. When we flare the ribs, or when the egg is open in the front, we lose the thoracic contact in the previous neutral spine dowel/broomstick example.

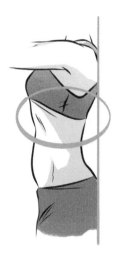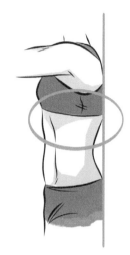

FIGURE 4.19 RIB FLARE

We can use this same concept to find neutral spine while lying on our back, in the supine position on a bed or the ground. When we lie on our back with our knees bent (in the hook-lying position) the same three points of the spine should be contacting the surface we are lying on. And, in neutral pelvis, there will be a small space to slide a hand between the ground and our lumbar spine. Note that the thorax point would not touch the ground if the ribs are flared. When we achieve awareness of our posture and centered trunk alignment, we can build upon this foundation and learn to recruit the muscles responsible for maintaining this zone. Centered alignment provides an optimal environment for coordinated and sustainable co-contraction of the core muscles.[40]

Passive Connective Tissue

Before we shift into a chapter solely about muscles, let's take a moment to note the tissues in between muscles and bones that also contribute to the stability of the spine. Specifically, let's look at the connective tissue structures: tendons, ligaments, and fascia. Tendons are cords of fibrous collagen tissue attaching a muscle to a bone; ligaments attach bones to bones. Connective tissue can be categorized as passive or active. Tendons and ligaments are passive tissue, meaning their protein cells do not possess contractile properties (while muscles do possess active contractile proteins).

Fascia

Fascia is considered passive tissue and is technically defined as "a thin casing of connective tissue that surrounds and holds every organ, blood vessel, bone, nerve fiber and muscle in place."[41] This system covers the body. "Fascia is generally defined as connective tissue composed of irregularly arranged collagen fibers, in contrast to the regularly arranged collagen fibers seen in tendons, ligaments or aponeurotic sheets."[42] I think of fascia as sheets of plastic wrap hugging and compartmentalizing organs and tissue bundles. Zügel and colleagues posit that "The fascial system builds a three-dimensional continuum of soft, collagen-containing, loose and dense fibrous connective tissue that permeates the body and enables all body systems to operate in an integrated manner."[43]

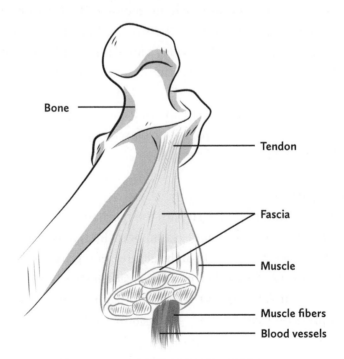

FIGURE 4.20 CONNECTIVE TISSUE STRUCTURE

Fascia can also be considered a transition tissue. In addition to providing internal structure, it has nerves that make it almost as sensitive as skin. "When stressed, it tightens up."[44] There is emerging research that suggests that, mechanically, fascia can act as both a liquid and a solid.[45] Tom Myers, the developer of the concept "anatomy trains,"[46] is famous for "turning his scalpel sideways" after developing a game for his students to play while teaching fascial anatomy at the Rolf Institute. His idea that there are 12 continuous fascial lines which run through the body is a paradigm shift in the way movement and body work professionals think about the function and anatomy of fascia.[47] Zügel et al. note that "Fascial tissues deserve more detailed attention in the field of sports medicine."[48] We are learning more about how fascia responds and adapts to mechanical overload, performance, and pain. When nerve pain receptors become enmeshed in fascial densification and fibrosis, deep fascia can be a source of pain.[49]

Fascia provides stability and function to the core. "Current evidence suggests that the muscles and fascia of the lumbo-pelvic region play a significant role in musculoskeletal function as well as continence and respiration."[50] "Passive...resting myofascial tension is present in the body and provides a low-level stabilizing component to help maintain balanced postures. This property [is] called *human resting myofascial tone* (HRMT)."[51] This resting myofascial tone's "passive role in helping to maintain balanced postures is supported by biomechanical principles of myofascial elasticity, tension, stress, stiffness, and tensegrity."[52]

Tensegrity

Tensegrity and biotensegrity are the mechanisms by which kinesiologists now suggest that fascia supports human resting myofascial tone or tension.[53, 54, 55, 56] In architecture, tensegrity is the characteristic property of a stable three-dimensional structure consisting of members under tension that are contiguous, and members under compression that are not.[57] At its simplest, tensegrity is a physics principle whereby objects push and pull against each other, creating opposing forces which cause an object to be held in place. The term was coined by Buckminster Fuller in the 1960s as a contraction of "tensional integrity."[58] It is the principle by which the children's toy shown in Figure 4.21 expands back to its original shape after compression. Fascia helps give our material body resting tone. The passive core includes fascia, and fascia is a transitional tissue between the passive bony core and the active muscular core.

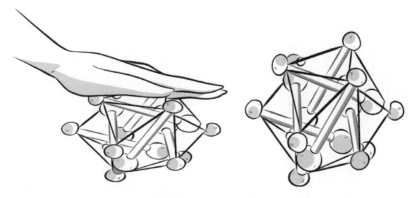

FIGURE 4.21 TENSEGRITY

5

THE MUSCULAR CORE

Core Muscles

I define the muscular core as all the muscles that attach to the bony core. In the previous chapter, we noted that the bony core is the cylinder of scaffolding made by our skeleton when we remove our arms, legs, and skull. *All* the muscles that attach to this trunk cylinder are considered core muscles.

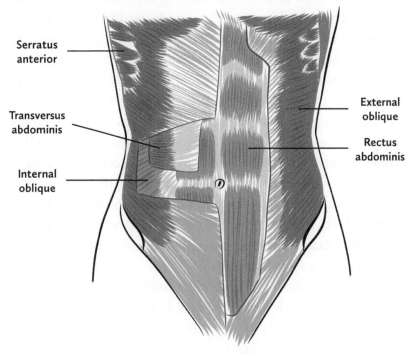

FIGURE 5.1 THE MUSCULAR CORE

The core muscles provide the mechanical support necessary to move a limb.[1] In other words, the core muscles stabilize the trunk cylinder to allow our arms, legs, and head to move freely in space. "At higher forces, the degrees of freedom of the system are reduced to promote inter-joint coordination and stability at the expense of flexibility."[2] Basically, we are constantly balancing stability and flexibility. Just like in yoga, we are seeking the balance between stability and ease, which is the definition of *asana*.

Proximal Stability Yields Distal Mobility

One definition of *core stability* is "the ability to control the position and motion of the trunk over the pelvis to allow optimum production, transfer and control of force and motion to the terminal segment in integrated athletic activities."[3] In order for this to occur, the trunk muscles need to coordinate or *co-contract*. In the core, "Muscle co-contraction, the simultaneous activation of antagonistic and agonistic muscles, plays an important role in...stabilizing [the] lumbar spine."[4] In other words, the antagonistic and agonistic, or opposing, muscles work together and provide spinal stability prior to moving a limb. "Normal, efficient motion and muscle activation are believed to occur in a proximal-to-distal sequence."[5] When the core muscles in the trunk are functioning normally, the result is "proximal stability for distal mobility, a proximal to distal patterning of generation of force, and the creation of interactive moments that move and protect distal joints."[6]

It is the trunk or core muscles which provide that *proximal stability for distal mobility* and better limb, or distal, performance.[7, 8] "Core stability is an extension of the closed kinetic chain theory, recognizing that...a strong core is required to stabilize the body so our limbs can be forceful lever arms."[9]

In healthy populations, certain trunk muscles have been shown to spontaneously co-activate in advance of limb movement.[10] These are: the pelvic floor muscles,[11] transverse abdominis muscle (TVA),[12, 13] multifidus,[14] respiratory diaphragm muscle (RD),[15, 16] scapular stabilizers,[17] and glottis.[18] They "wink" or "pre-contract" when we simply prepare to move a limb![19] Voluntary movement of the upper limb is preceded by postural movements occurring in the lower limbs and the pelvis.[20] This is also termed "feed-forward" contraction in the literature.[21] Conversely, *uncoordinated* core muscle action in the pelvic floor, deep abdominals, and respiratory diaphragm muscles have been seen in low back pain and pelvic girdle issues.[22, 23, 24, 25, 26, 27, 28] The understanding that trunk muscle activity can be altered in patients with pain perpetuated the idea that rehabilitation professionals could retrain these muscles to help with their symptoms.[29]

We have to be careful, though, as we learn more about the integrated nature of the body and its inseparable layers. There is no one-size-fits-all treatment. We cannot make causal assumptions that certain muscles are more important for stabilization of the spine than other muscles. While McCook et al. provide some evidence supporting the contribution of TrA to lumbo-pelvic stability,[30] isolating one core muscle, such as the transverse abdominis alone, is not a solution. Furthermore, evidence that core stabilization exercises alleviate back pain just does not exist.[31] Exercise is beneficial for chronic pain. "However, the claim that core stability exercise is one of the most effective options for low-back pain is without merit and clearly lacks supporting evidence."[32] And, in a systematic review with meta-analysis, "There is strong evidence stabilisation exercises [for low back pain] are not more effective than any other form of active exercise in the long term...and further research is unlikely to considerably alter this conclusion."[33] "Despite a decade of extensive research in this area, it is difficult to see what contribution CS had to the understanding and care of patients suffering from back pain."[34]

While further study might be necessary, "What is known is that trunk muscle activation is adjusted to meet stability demands, which highlights that the central nervous system closely monitors threats to spine stability."[35] We will discuss the threat to the nervous system more in Chapter 6, The Breathing Core. Meanwhile, with this lack of causal evidence in mind, Reeves and colleagues (2019) argue "for a more contemporary and broadened view of stability that integrates interdisciplinary knowledge in order to capture the complexity of back pain."[36]

Let's not confuse static stability with dynamic stability. Physical therapy traditionally taught static pelvic floor and transverse abdominis muscle contraction as a response to acute back pain. This is also sometimes taught in a "fast flow" or physically rigorous yoga class. This might work as a learning strategy for muscle engagement, but we are always breathing, and the core muscles are always moving. We can still achieve dynamic core stability. "If [one] can really trust the inhalation and allow for that natural movement of the diaphragm and the pelvic floor, that breath in by itself will create the stability [one needs] for [the] spine."[37] In order to understand the whole organism, we will examine some individual muscle groups of the core.

When I am assessing core muscle coordination in clients, I observe how all the trunk muscles are working in symphony (or not) during a given movement. Intervention is always customized, based on how an individual presents. When there is a movement pattern problem, I hone in on how the *anticipatory* core muscles are firing. Are the forces and timing of the muscles coordinated and appropriate for the task? As noted, the pelvic floor, deep abdominals, and respiratory diaphragm muscles are *uncoordinated* in the presence of lumbo-pelvic disorders. When I observe this in the clinic, I find it useful to help clients regain control of these muscles as part of their rehabilitation program. Additionally, I include the scapular stabilizing muscles and glottis in the anticipatory core muscle group. I define this entire group as the *sustainable core muscles.*

Sustainable Core Muscles

When I observe a client move in any chosen task, I look at the coordination of their sustainable core muscles, which include the:

- pelvic floor muscles
- deep abdominal muscles
- scapular stabilizing muscles
- glottis/pharyngeal muscles
- respiratory diaphragm muscle.

These are postural muscles, part of the group that holds our skeleton up against gravity all day. Postural muscles are mainly endurance muscles or contain a higher percentage of slow-twitch muscle fibers. This implies that they don't require as much energy to contract—hence the term "sustainable." Their minimal "job" is to hold up our bones against gravity. This group of core muscles automatically engage to support trunk stability in anticipation of limb movement or disturbance. It has been suggested in the literature that "Coordinated retraining [of] diaphragmatic, deep abdominal and PFM function could improve symptoms and quality of life" in patients with urinary stress incontinence.[38] We will discuss the special role of the respiratory diaphragm muscle in Chapter 6, and I will support and discuss my argument for including the glottis and scapular stabilizers in this group shortly. Again, we are looking at the coordination of the orchestra and how the muscles are co-contracting to meet the demands of the given task. Before we can look at the entire symphony of the core muscular system, let's examine its players.

Pelvic Floor Muscles
Healthy Pelvic Floor Muscles
The muscles on the inferior bowl of the pelvis make up the pelvic floor muscles (PFM). They comprise the dynamic muscular "floor" of the bony core cylinder.[39] "The pelvic floor muscles (PFM) are part of the trunk stability mechanism. Their function is interdependent with other muscles of this system. They also contribute to continence, elimination, sexual arousal and intra-abdominal pressure."[40] PFM are "The anatomic structures that prevent incontinence and genital organ prolapse on increases in abdominal pressure during daily activities [and] include sphincteric and supportive systems."[41] The muscles support the pelvic organs and abdominal viscera (assisting with the support that keeps our organs snug) and they help with continence (keeping our wastes in until we choose to expel them).

In both sexes, the pelvic floor is comprised of a number of muscles which are organized into superficial and deep muscle layers. I tell clients that I won't test them on the muscle names, but I like to introduce their proper names at the outset. The *superficial muscle layer* contains the external sphincters (anal and urethral), ischiocavernosus, bulbospongiosus, the superficial transverse perineal muscles, and the perineal body. The middle layer consists of the deep transverse perineal muscles, fascia, and membranes. The *deep pelvic floor muscles* consist of the levator ani (which is a combination of the pubococcygeus and iliococcygeus muscles) and the coccygeus muscles.[42] The obturator internus and piriformis muscles which cover the pelvic floor *and* the hip are considered part of the deep layer.[43]

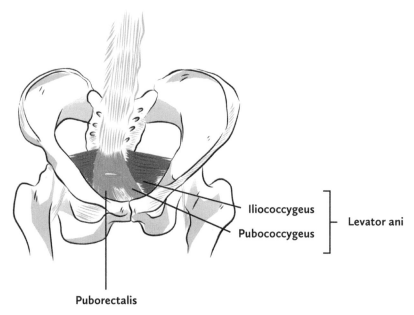

Iliococcygeus

Pubococcygeus

Levator ani

Puborectalis

FIGURE 5.2 PELVIC FLOOR MUSCLES

Contraction of PFM precedes coughing or sneezing to maintain continence and to protect the pelvic floor from the sudden increase of intra-abdominal pressure (IAP).[44, 45] IAP is the force in the abdomen created during normal movements like lifting, bending, carrying, and straining. The pelvic floor muscles help keep the pelvic organs (bladder, bowels, and uterus, if present) in position during movement.

At rest, the pelvic floor muscles have a normal tone somewhere in the midrange of motion, where they keep our pelvic and abdominal contents snug and continent. In other words, the optimal resting state of a muscle is not loose, disconnected, or "flapping in the wind." There is a little bit of tension keeping the muscle connected, but it is not normal for the muscle to be fully contracted all the time, either. This normal midrange tone increases just before we cough or sneeze, or move a limb.[46,47,48] Interestingly, one study implied that, *in vivo* (or "in real life"), the pelvic floor muscles are shaped like a dome, not a sling or basin as we see in cadaver subjects and anatomy books.[49] This is controversial and would imply that the domes of the respiratory diaphragm muscle and the pelvic floor are actually parallel to each other. Experienced internal pelvic health therapists disagree, noting that a dome-shaped pelvic bowl might imply a hypertonic pelvic floor muscle system.

The physical medicine literature includes the pelvic floor musculature as having an important role in respiration, as a key player in the generation of intra-abdominal pressure, and as an accessory expiratory muscle.[50,51] The degree of exhalation force changes the recruitment of the PFM. In one study that looked at the degree of PFM contraction with forced expiration, researchers found that less is more. "Minimal forced expiration effort resulted in the most consistent PF cranial-ventral displacement with vaginal squeeze pressure."[52]

We cannot separate the coordination of the pelvic floor muscles from breathing or trunk stability; they happen together. The superficial and deep layers anticipate and respond differently depending on the task. "The deep layer was more tightly modulated with respiration than the superficial layer, but activation of the superficial layer was greater during maximal/submaximal occluded respiratory efforts and earlier during cough."[53]

PFM Influencers

Just as we can't uncouple the pelvic floor muscles from the orchestra of the core muscles, there are other factors influencing the recruitment of the PFMs.[54] Tissue damage,[55,56,57,58] hormones,[59,60,61] emotional health[62,63] (stress, anxiety/depression,[64,65,66,67] or fear[68]), breathing patterns, and lumbo-pelvic alignment all influence the response and recruitment of the pelvic floor muscles.[69]

Alignment and posture influence the *length–tension relationship* of the PFM recruitment.[70, 71, 72] The length–tension relationship of a muscle basically describes the amount of tension that is produced by a muscle as a feature of its length. In other words, under isometric conditions, the maximal force produced or measured will be different as the muscle lengthens or shortens. Muscle length affects muscle tension by increasing the resting length of the sarcomere—the functional muscle cell unit—which increases the distance that the muscle cell filaments can slide over each other and, thus, develop tension or force development.[73]

PFM activity varies with the lumbar curve and different sitting postures in healthy women.[74] Functionally, the pelvic floor muscles have the optimal length–tension potential for full range of motion contraction and relaxation in an upright, neutral lumbar position.[75] In a study by Capson et al. which measured PFM activity in various postures and tasks, their results "clearly indicate that changes in lumbo-pelvic posture influence both the contractility of the PFMs and the amount of vaginal pressure generated during static postures and during dynamic tasks."[76] "Lumbo-pelvic posture does not, however, appear to have a significant effect on the timing of PFM activation during coughing or load-catching tasks."[77] Again, it's multifactorial; alignment is just one influence.

Compromised PFM

When the function and integrity of the pelvic floor muscles are compromised, "the results lead to many of the problems seen by clinicians."[78] These problems can include incontinence, and pelvic organ prolapse.[79] Often times people don't know that their PFM are compromised and they don't seek help until they experience symptoms of discomfort or incontinence. The relationship between pelvic pain and compromised PFM activity is tricky. Research supports "the hypothesis that pelvic floor muscle dysfunction is present among women with lumbo-pelvic pain."[80] We shouldn't overlook musculoskeletal dysfunction as a possible factor in chronic pelvic pain and properly designed studies are "urgently needed to determine the true effectiveness of treatments for pelvic musculoskeletal pain."[81] One investigation attempted to look into the common factors of chronic pelvic pain in women, and found that there might be similar postural, breathing, or movement patterns, but the causes are still not clear and further investigation is warranted.[82] The causes of a compromised pelvic floor are individual and multifactorial.

For older women with pelvic floor symptoms, menopause is associated with impaired responsiveness of involuntary PFM contractions to sudden intra-abdominal pressure rise, but not correlated with decreased voluntary PFM contractions.[83] In other words, menopause is not associated with decreased PFM concentric strength. Yet incontinence in young, highly fit, nulliparous women is present. In one study, 28 percent of elite college varsity female athletes reported incontinence.[84] We can infer that the elite athletes' core muscles are probably strong, so what's going on?

While it is common (but not normal!) for menopausal people to have weakened pelvic floor muscles and experience some incontinence, why are one in four college athletes peeing their pants? Again, the causes of a dysfunctional pelvic floor are multifactorial and not necessarily related to age. "Pelvic floor dysfunction can also involve the development of hypertonic, dysfunctional muscles."[85] Not only does strength play a role in a functional pelvic floor, so does muscle tissue suppleness, flexibility, and coordination of the pelvic floor muscles with the other core muscles.

We can't always associate PFM *weakness* with dysfunction. Strengthening the pelvic floor in isolation, or practicing Kegel exercises, is not necessarily the best treatment for incontinence,[86, 87, 88, 89, 90, 91, 92, 93, 94] and could make situations worse in some cases![95] Incontinence can be seen with weak pelvic floor muscles, but also with muscles that are overactive, or are less resilient.

To be clear, we cannot determine if the PFM muscles are overactive, underactive, hypertonic, hypotonic, or even weak or strong, without an internal assessment (manual/digital or with an EMG) performed by a trained and licensed health care professional. We can, however, make certain inferences about whether the PFM are functioning properly or not, by understanding the normal sequence of muscle timing and coordination in a healthy muscular core.

In order to maintain continence, the pelvic floor and transverse abdominis muscles coordinate to maintain appropriate intra-abdominal pressure and bladder neck length. A submaximal PFM contraction is more effective at holding our urine in than a maximal contraction. A licensed and trained practitioner can use perineal ultrasound to ensure bladder-neck effective pelvic floor contraction and help clients with overactive bladder and incontinence symptoms by actively integrating the submaximal "pelvic floor contraction into daily life and individual incontinence triggering activities."[96] Women with stress urinary incontinence recruit their muscles differently during coughing than those without incontinence.[97] Women with urine leakage during coughing demonstrated altered core muscle activation patterns, difficulty performing voluntary contraction of the PFM, and a tendency to substitute other muscles. The SUI "may be related to delays in force generation rather than PFM weakness."[98]

One study that investigated trunk muscle activity and static balance tasks in women with and without SUI demonstrated that "women with SUI have decreased balance ability compared to continent women" whether or not their bladder was full or empty. This suggests that women with incontinence have increased PF and abdominal muscle activity associated with postural perturbations. It is proposed that "Increased activity of the PF and trunk muscles in women with SUI may impair balance as a result of a reduced contribution of trunk movement to postural correction or compromised proprioceptive acuity."[99] As these findings show, we can't simply isolate one group of trunk muscles. The PFM work together as a symphony with the core muscles, and all the players matter.[100, 101, 102, 103, 104, 105]

PFM Rehabilitation

What does rehabilitation of the pelvic floor muscles mean in practical terms? Historically, clinicians have been telling women to do their Kegel exercises whenever they wait at a red light, but that may not be the best advice. Again, some pelvic floor issues are caused by weak pelvic floors, but this is only one factor to consider. In men and women, every muscle needs full available length and strength in order to respond to normal movements in life. The pelvic floor muscles are no exception. The functional length and strength of a muscle is dependent on the load of a task. For example, in a well-functioning pelvic floor, the muscles will "wink" or reflexively engage in antici- pation of lifting an object from the floor. If this object is a feather or pencil, the amount of force or contraction necessary to remain continent is minimal. However, if the object is a 15-pound squirming baby, the amount of force needed by the pelvic floor muscles is higher to maintain continence. If the pelvic floor muscles were in a state of healthy resting tone prior to lifting the baby, then there is enough available range of motion for the muscles to engage further prior to lifting the baby, while maintaining continence. However, in an overactive pelvic floor situation, the muscles are already shortened toward their end-range. In that case, there is limited range of motion for the muscles to contract further and there is not enough reserve range of motion to maintain closure. This person might "spring a leak" with the added pressure of the 15-pound load, because the pelvic floor muscles did not have enough available suppleness or potential resilience to maintain closure of the urethral openings. A good exam- ple of this is to compare the PFM muscles to the biceps muscle in the arm. If we walk around with our elbow bent all day, never lengthening the biceps muscle, our elbow function is markedly diminished.

Three theories exist to explain why retraining the PFM for treat- ing SUI is effective.[106] One idea is that abdominal muscle training indirectly strengthens the PFM; this is not supported in the literature. The other two ideas are supported by randomized controlled trials. The first is a behavioral construct where "women learn to consciously pre-contract the PFMs before and during increases in abdominal pressure (such as coughing, physical activity) to prevent leakage."[107] The second theory is that "strength training builds up long-lasting muscle volume and thus provides structural support," which has the "aim of changing neuromuscular function and morphology, thus making the PFM contraction automatic."[108] Both theories are supported by the "conscious competence learning theory" I will introduce in Chapter 7, The Mindful Core. The goal is to practice a new behavior to eventually make it automatic.

Should we practice Kegels or not? The answer is: "It depends." The American Urological Association advises avoiding pelvic floor strengthening exercises (Kegels) for treating interstitial cystitis/bladder pain syndrome where pelvic pain is present and PFM are overactive.[109] I pause here to offer some practical advice: if Kegels do not help, or if practicing them makes your situation worse, please discontinue the practice and seek the assistance of a licensed health care provider who is trained in internal pelvic floor assessments. Again, every muscle requires optimal length and strength for best function and available resilience, and strength alone does not translate into function. There are effective alternative approaches to PFM dysfunctions.[110, 111, 112, 113, 114, 115, 116, 117, 118]

Pelvic floor muscle training (PFMT), which includes *relaxing* and engaging the PFM, is significantly more effective for SUI than no treatment or education alone. The findings of a 2018 Cochrane review of the research suggest "that PFMT could be included in first-line conservative management programmes for women with UI."[119] Furthermore, recommended treatment for pelvic floor hypertonic disorders "typically involves biofeedback techniques, teaching relaxation, or reverse Kegels,"[120] performed by a specially trained pelvic floor clinician. It is perfectly safe to attempt to relax (and engage) the pelvic floor muscles on your own, and I encourage you to try the reverse Kegel exercise presented in Chapter 11 of this book for your own awareness and calibration of your PFM awareness. You do not need to be trained in internal pelvic floor muscle assessment to observe or practice any technique offered in this book.

I encourage you to take a moment right now to explore this information in your own body. In Chapter 4, we learned how to tuck our pelvis (posterior pelvic tilt and lumbar flexion), find neutral pelvis/spine, and how to extend our pelvis (anterior pelvic tilt and lumbar extension). Try performing a reverse Kegel and a light pelvic floor contraction in each of the three positions. Note if one position is easier than another, or makes it more difficult to contract or relax the pelvic floor muscles. Generally, the best length–tension relationship of the PFM is in neutral pelvis.

Pelvic floor awareness is certainly a first treatment choice in the clinic when I am assessing someone with a complaint of incontinence or pelvic pain. Clinically, I find that those who have trouble relaxing the PFM are usually harboring chronic pain or tension, and that their muscle coordination has gone "offline" in what may have initially been an effective protection response. The body is adaptive and resilient. Remember, the muscles of the pelvic floor do not act alone.

Rehabilitation of pelvic floor dysfunction is usually focused only on the PFM, and in most programs training of other parts of the core muscles is often neglected. Even though it is a cost-effective and viable treatment option, PFM training is often underutilized.[121] "Even as we improve our basic science understanding of common central neuro-logic mechanisms underlying persistent pain, our current research strategy into pelvic pain management must include musculoskeletal dysfunction."[122] The retraining of correct patterns of core muscle recruitment with diaphragmatic breathing, deep abdominal muscles, and PFMT exercises has been reported as a successful approach to treat female SUI and has been implemented by some therapists.[123, 124]

When retraining the PFM, rehabilitation programs need to take all this into account as we cannot separate the parts from the whole organism. An integrative pelvic floor rehabilitation program that includes submaximal PFM co-contraction with the TVA is highly effective for reducing stress urinary incontinence and overactive bladder symptoms.[125] Pelvic floor muscle rehabilitation programs should be individualized, and the treatment goal is to normalize the intra-abdominal pressure with co-contraction of the PFM and the deep abdominal muscles, especially the transverse abdominis muscle.

Coordination of PFM with Abdominal Muscles

Deep *abdominal* muscle activity is also a normal response to pelvic floor muscle exercise in subjects with no symptoms of pelvic floor muscle dysfunction.[126, 127, 128] One can engage their abdominal muscles without contracting the pelvic floor muscles. However, the abdominal muscles respond to PFM engagement. An EMG study determined that "It was not possible [for the subjects in the study] to contract the pelvic floor effectively while maintaining relaxation of the deep abdominal muscles."[129] I use this tidbit in the clinic often to externally assess or screen clients' ability to perform a pelvic floor contraction. I have the client place their hands (or with consent, I place mine) on their lower abdomen and ask them to engage their PFM (or in lay-terms, perform a "Kegel"). If there is no response in the deep abdominal muscles, breath holding, or an *increase* in abdominal circumference (pooching out), I might begin to suspect inefficient pelvic floor muscle function. Please note that there is no evidence for the opposite scenario: strengthening the abdominal muscles alone does *not* facilitate PFM contraction.[130] One doesn't have to be trained in internal pelvic assessments to get an idea of how someone's pelvic floor might be functioning (or not). A coordinated recruitment pattern of core muscles is needed for spine stabilization. It is not about the strength but the *sequence* of motor unit recruitment of all core muscles, and the functional co-contraction between the transverse abdominis, diaphragm, and pelvic floor muscles.[131, 132, 133, 134]

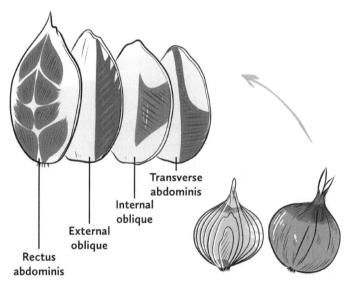

FIGURE 5.3 THE LAYERS OF THE ABDOMINAL MUSCLES

Transverse Abdominis Muscle
Healthy TVA

The second group of sustainable core muscles to consider are the deep abdominal muscles. The deepest, the transverse abdominis muscle, has a major role in lumbo-pelvic stability,[135] and traditionally the abdominal muscles are considered main players in the core muscle symphony.[136]

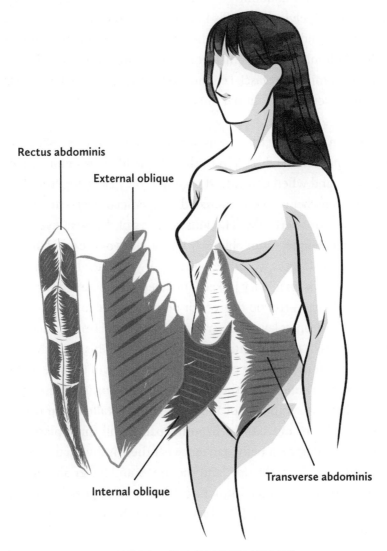

FIGURE 5.4 THE ABDOMINAL MUSCLES

The abdominal muscles, sometimes called the "abs," are four layers of muscles on the front of the trunk. All four have attachments to the pelvis and the ribs. The most superficial muscle, the rectus abdominis (RA), runs vertically from the fascia of the pubic bone to the sternum, or breastbone. The superficial rectus abdominis muscle does not have a direct role in lumbar stability. The three deeper layers (from superficial to deep) are the external obliques (EO), the internal obliques (IO), and the transverse abdominis (TVA). These three muscles not only span from the pelvis to the ribs like their superficial neighbor, but also wrap around to the sides of the trunk and have attachments to the thoracolumbar fascia, which connects to the spine and pelvis. It is because of this direct fascial connection to the spine and pelvis that these three deeper abdominal muscles have a role in lumbo-pelvic stability.

Functionally, these three muscles act as a team to stabilize the spine and pelvis. The direction of the muscle fibers is unique in all four layers, and when contracted together, they close together like tightening a basket weave. As noted, the superficial layer—the rectus abdominis—runs vertically. The muscle fibers of the next layer in— the external obliques—run obliquely on the sides of the trunk in the direction your fingers would be pointing if you placed your hands in pockets on an imaginary jacket. The fibers of the next layer—the internal obliques—run 90 degrees or perpendicular to the external obliques. The deepest layer—the transverse abdominis muscle fibers— runs transversely or horizontally across the trunk. This basket weave of abdominal muscles make up a significant portion of the side of the tin can we were building on the bony core scaffolding (see Figure 5.1).

Together, the symphony of abdominal muscles allows our pelvis, spine, and ribs to move or be fixed in space in all three planes of movement. Imagine a belly dancer, with their individual control of the left side, the right side, and the upper and lower abdominal muscles undulating and contracting. This is made possible by the "regional differentiation in [TVA] activity with challenges to postural control."[137]

Stabilizing the trunk is the most important function of abdominal muscles. Abdominal muscles can be categorized into two groups: the deep stabilizers and the superficial mobilizers. "The stabilizers include transverse abdominis (TrAb) and internal oblique (IO), and the mobilizers include [rectus abdominis] and [external obliques]. These muscles together are responsible for producing gross movement of trunk and pelvis."[138] I learned in school that in a healthy pelvis and spine, the deepest of these muscles—the transverse abdominis muscle—will contract in anticipation of a limb movement.[139, 140, 141] This is the same feedforward mechanism or anticipatory engagement that is observed in the pelvic floor muscles.[142] The deep abdominals are recruited before the superficial,[143] and the muscle tension should match the load and direction of the task.[144] Recall the example where the deep pelvic floor muscles will engage differently in anticipation of the load—picking up a pencil versus a heavy, moving baby. The same is true in the abdomen. "The coordination of limb movement and its associated 'anticipatory' postural response may not be limited to a single strategy and may vary, depending on the biomechanical contribution of the individual muscles to postural stability."[145] Trunk stability strategy is individual and "results from highly coordinated muscle activation patterns involving many muscles, and...the recruitment patterns must continually change, depending on the task."[146]

Healthy engagement of the TVA feels like a deep sheet of elastic fabric that is recoiling inwardly, after it has been stretched away horizontally from the belly button. The TVA can lose its tonic function in chronic low back pain, and it has been suggested that it should be trained separately from the other trunk muscles to contract tonically but not at a constant level.[147] Just like the pelvic floor muscles, the normal resting tone of the abdominal muscles is a range somewhere in between hypotonic (floppy) and hypertonic (too rigid or overactive). Healthy core muscles hang out in the midrange of tone and will contract to anticipate limb movement.[148] For these reasons, the sequence, timing, and degree of contraction of the transverse abdominis receives a lot of attention in musculoskeletal rehabilitation for trunk stabilization. EMG studies suggest that "Perhaps the main action responsible for raising the intra-abdominal pressure [to protect the intervertebral discs from compression load] is supplied by the transverse abdominis muscle."[149]

It is quite common and useful for rehabilitation and movement professionals to retrain the transverse abdominis muscle to properly engage before moving a limb in any movement. A common progression of lumbo-pelvic stabilization exercises, offered by physical therapist Shirley Sahrmann, is still used and validated today.[150] I offer the directions for variations of some of these exercises in the final chapter of this book.

Compromised TVA

I also learned in PT school that TVA response is altered in back pain.[151, 152, 153, 154, 155, 156, 157, 158, 159, 160, 161] Pinto and colleagues report that "Neutral lumbar posture can facilitate an increase in thickness of the [TVA] muscle while performing a leg task...however, this effect was not observed for this muscle in patients with LBP."[162] While we have established that the TVA responds differently when LBP is reported, the relationship between trunk muscle strength and lumbar pain is still debatable. The "association between abdominal endurance and low back pain in athletes (including dancers) is weak."[163] And trunk "muscle strength is also a poor predictor of risk for development of LBP in athletes."[164] One study compared the results of the balance-dexterity task in people with healthy backs versus those with recurrent low back pain and found "Persons with recurrent LBP exhibited more dissociated trunk motion during the task than did back-healthy controls, which was related to reduced deep trunk muscle activity relative to more superficial trunk muscles."[165] Like the PFM, in a compromised system, sometimes the superficial abdominal muscle layers are recruited while the deep layers remain "offline." More research on this theory observed "increased superficial trunk muscle activity in subjects with chronic LBP during walking"[166] which supports the idea that the superficial trunk muscle activity reflects an underlying guarding mechanism. So, the evidence of altered abdominal muscle recruitment in LBP cannot be causal or correlated, but "the relationship between co-contraction and back pain development may actually be circular, in that it is both causal and adaptive."[167]

We need to move beyond a mechanistic view and biomechanics.[168] We can't assume "that the directional invariant bilateral feedforward response of transversus abdominis is acting as a corset stabilizer and is the normal pattern for all spinal perturbations."[169] We should take care and be careful "in the interpretation that all other activation patterns represent motor control dysfunction and that this can be translated into a mechanical inference that these individuals have less than optimal core stability. The evidence is just not there."[170]

As I have mentioned, our bodies are resilient and adaptive. Perhaps this overactivity of the superficial abdominal muscles "initially predisposes to pain development, following which co-contraction further increases in an attempt to alleviate the pain, and the cycle perpetuates."[171] Again, we are looking at how the whole symphony of the trunk muscles work together in the entire canister, and this is task-dependent.

The abdominal muscles receive a lot of attention in the pregnant and postpartum bodies. Just take a moment to marvel at how much these muscles and surrounding tissues stretch to accommodate a growing baby and uterus to full term!

> Pregnancy-related diastasis rectus abdominis is a term used to describe the process wherein the connective tissue strip down the mid-line of the abdomen, the linea alba, widens and thins to accommodate the growing baby. This natural physiological process has been reported to occur in 100% of pregnant women.[172]

Since this happens in all full-term pregnancies, it should be considered normal, and a functional postpartum goal should include regaining the various length–tension responses required for the loads of daily tasks.

However, the old definition of pregnancy-related tissue thinning and stretching at the vertical midline of the anterior trunk included the rectus abdominis muscle physically separating at the midline.[173]

And, according to the old paradigm, if this situation impaired the function of the trunk, the condition was called *diastasis recti abdominis* (DRA). The rehabilitation focus used to be placed on "closing the gap" and the old consensus was that any gap wider than two finger-widths was considered worth closing. Physical therapists traditionally have prescribed exercises targeting the TVA as a method for reducing inter-recti distance (IRD) in the postpartum population.[174] Some studies show that abdominal drawing in exercises targeted at the deep abdominals may actually *widen* the intersection distance,[175, 176] and that certain exercises could improve the tensile response of the linea alba without increasing the IRD.[177]

The paradigm is shifting as we learn more about the body's return to activity after pregnancy. We are becoming more interested in restoring the functional tension in the abdominal tissues and whether the body can maintain tension in the linea alba throughout an exercise or task. "There is a shift from using words such as 'split' or 'separated' towards simply describing the physiological process of linea alba widening and thinning that occurs during pregnancy. This shift in vocabulary helps to reduce fear associated with having 'split' muscles."[178] The "doming" of the rectus abdominis muscle might be a protective response and the new paradigm understands "that doming operates within a continuum [which] allows for a more individualized assessment of pressure management."[179] "In the cases where doming appears to be at the patient's end limit, we can modify exercise parameters such as breath, posture, [and] core engagement... to assess if their doming can come down from the extremes."[180]

Lee and Hodges[181] propose a hypothesis that contraction of the PFM with co-activation of the TVA may tighten the linea alba, and hence be important for the function of the abdominal wall. So again, we are looking at how the pelvic floor and abdominal muscles are working together to create global trunk stability for the functional tasks at hand. In the case of DRA, we are interested in the functional tension of the trunk to respond to and manage intra-abdominal pressure. This can look different in different bodies. Traditionally, we've looked at the drawing in of the deep abdominal muscles as a healthy function of pressure management.

When the rectus abdominis muscle (the *superficial* abdominal muscle; it's the one that does not contribute to lumbar stabilization) contracts by itself, it appears to dome or "pooch." This is not a problematic contraction strategy for picking up a pencil if a client has no reports of pain or dysfunction. But if a person with DRA also reports pain, pelvic organ prolapse, or incontinence, the best way we currently know how to help them restore trunk support is to support the entire trunk and recruit more of the abdominal muscle team. This means they should co-contract the PFM and deep abdominal muscles *with* the RA. This support can be *external*, with a brace or their own hands, and/or *internal*, by restoring the coordination of the PFM with the abdominal muscles in preparation for, and during, a task. In all new exercises that involve increased load, we want to safely explore the body's control and reaction. We just watch for end-range recruitment. "Each patient will have their own range of doming/bulging and it is useful to assess where, in that continuum, the patient's doming exists."[182] Further, it should be noted that "Any exercise and/or movement can be used as a goal and can be broken down into its progressive components. The patient can advance through the levels allowing them to gain confidence in their abilities."[183]

The Parallel Pelvic Floor Muscles and the Diaphragm

Recall that the PFM work synergistically with other muscle groups.[184, 185, 186, 187, 188, 189] The transverse abdominis muscle responds to pelvic floor muscle contractions, and the pelvic floor muscles are parallel to the domes of the respiratory diaphragm muscle. The pelvic floor muscles, posture, and respiration are interconnected, and we can't uncouple breathing from the core muscles.[190] We are always breathing, and even when we are sleeping we are constantly moving! The RD and PFM move in tandem like a piston.[191]

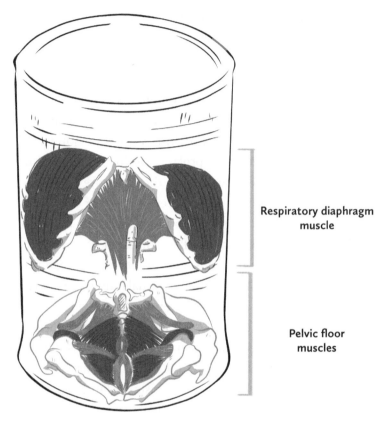

FIGURE 5.5 PELVIC FLOOR MUSCLES AND RESPIRATORY DIAPHRAGM

When we inhale, the domes of the respiratory diaphragm muscle flatten. This pushes the contents of the abdomen (mostly the intestines and pelvic organs) down onto the pelvic floor. And on the exhale, the pelvic floor muscles and respiratory diaphragm muscle recoil to their initial shapes simultaneously. The RD and PFM move in parallel, like a piston engine. This is why, initially, I cue the relaxation of the pelvic floor muscles with the inhalation and, when warranted, the engagement with the exhalation. The other reason is that the PFM are accessory exhaling muscles, so I like to retrain them to get back "online" to contract with the exhalation and relax on the inhalation. Studies have borne this out. "Both layers of PFM are activated during both inspiration and expiration, but with a bias to greater activation in expiratory tasks/phases."[192] In life, our pelvic floor and respiratory diaphragm muscles are always moving and adapting to our position in space. Our bodies also exert normal force and stability during inhalation—it is okay to lift a baby while inhaling! When helping someone regain control over tight or weak PFM, in a compromised system, I find that beginning with breath awareness coordinated with pelvic floor muscle awareness is a fabulous entry point.

Respiratory Diaphragm Muscle

The primary breathing muscle is our respiratory diaphragm muscle (RD). "Except in cases of paralysis, the diaphragm is always used for breathing."[193] "The diaphragm is the main muscle of inspiration, and is responsible for generating the majority of inspiratory airflow."[194] The diaphragm muscle contains about 55 percent of type 1 (slow twitch/endurance/aerobic) muscle fibers and about 45 percent of type 2 fibers (fast twitch/power generating/anaerobic)[195] making it an extremely fatigue resistant muscle. It is the key to a sustainable core. "When its muscle fibers are activated in isolation, they shorten, the dome of the diaphragm descends, pleural [lung] pressure...falls, and abdominal pressure...rises."[196] The word diaphragm comes from the Greek roots *dia* (through) and *phrágma*, meaning "fence" (partition or wall). The RD is the physical partition between the abdomen and the thorax. The muscle itself looks like a two-domed mushroom, parachute, or umbrella. It has a central tendon (like the stem of a mushroom or the pole of an umbrella) which arises from the lumbar vertebrae and the edges of the domes attach to the inside of the rib cage, along the rims of the lower ribs. Even at rest, the rib cage expands "because the diaphragm is capable of creating chest as well as belly movement."[197]

In development:

The diaphragm attains its position in the transverse plane between four to six months after birth, and costal breathing is fully established at six-months. Once the position of the diaphragm is established it contributes to the development of stability of the spine and core, allowing the baby to roll, crawl, sit, stand, and begin to walk.[198]

The respiratory diaphragm:

> can be considered as two separate muscles consisting of the crural and costal diaphragms. The costal diaphragm originates primarily from the ribs, and the crural diaphragm from the lumbar vertebra, as two pillars (right and left crura, or "legs"). The esophageal hiatus is formed primarily by the right crus.[199]

Kinesiologists readily relate to the diaphragm as a respiratory muscle. "However, gastrointestinal physiologists are becoming increasingly aware of the value of this muscle in helping to stop gastric contents from refluxing into the oesophagus."[200]

The crural diaphragm has two functions, respiratory and gastrointestinal.[201] The esophagus, or the digestive tube in the throat, passes right through the RD muscle, and the lower esophageal sphincter is positioned at the level of the RD. If the RD is tight, the esophageal tube can get compressed, and this narrowing can be associated with acid reflux. Furthermore, "Patients with chronic low back pain appear to have both abnormal position and a steeper slope of the diaphragm."[202] It has also been revealed that "Diaphragm weakness, a consequence of diaphragm dysfunction and atrophy, is common in the ICU and associated with serious clinical consequences."[203] In other words, the respiratory diaphragm muscle is so important that I remind clients that, during exercise, "breathing is mandatory."

Just like the pelvic floor muscles and the transverse abdominis muscle, the respiratory diaphragm muscle also spontaneously co-activates in advance of limb movement[204] and is part of postural and trunk stability.[205, 206] And just like the TVA and PFM, RD coordination is sometimes altered in subjects with sacroiliac pain. It is a muscle just like any other, and it will respond to situations optimally if it has full length and strength. One way to lengthen the RD is to *stretch* it with a voluntary, deep breath, specifically a long, soft *inhalation*.

Some practitioners call breaths that specifically expand the length of the fibers of the RD a "diaphragmatic breath." But that is a pet peeve of a lot of clinicians, because *all* breathing is diaphragmatic (except in cases of paralysis).

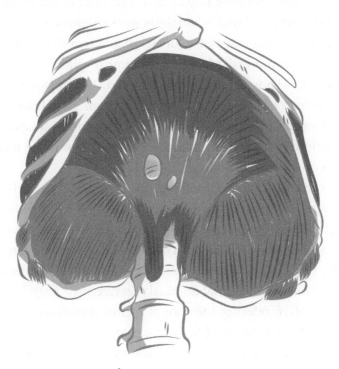

FIGURE 5.6 THE RESPIRATORY DIAPHRAGM

According to Nelson (2012), it is important to include diaphragmatic breathing with functional movement programs, as the diaphragm is the foundation of core stability.[207] As technology improves, magnetic resonance imaging (MRI) studies can be performed to analyze muscle function in real time. In one such study, Kolar et al. (2009) looked at diaphragm movement during tidal breathing synchronized with spirometry. Their small sample size confirmed "that the function of the diaphragm is not only respiratory but also postural and can be voluntarily controlled."[208] "The neurological control of breathing shows high levels of neuroplasticity as shown by its ability to adapt to a wide range of internal and external conditions."[209] This means, thankfully, that the RD responds and adapts to change, and we can exercise it.

The diaphragm muscle provides core stability by increasing intra-abdominal pressure. Some studies have indicated that people with sacroiliac pain have impaired recruitment of the diaphragm and pelvic floor.[210, 211] And, when the body encounters increased ventilation, challenges may cause further diaphragm dysfunction and lead to more compressive loads on the lumbar spine.[212] Akuthota et al. conclude: "Thus, diaphragmatic breathing techniques may be an important part of a core-strengthening program."[213] Additionally, the pelvic floor musculature is co-activated with transversus abdominis contraction[214] and the diaphragm and pelvic floor move together during coughing and breathing.[215]

We can't separate the functional interactions between the TVA, diaphragm, and pelvic floor muscles.[216] The abdominal muscles work synergistically with the respiratory muscles,[217, 218, 219] the pelvic floor muscles work synergistically with posture and respiratory muscles,[220] and the respiratory diaphragm muscle is intimately involved with posture control and intra-abdominal pressure.[221, 222, 223, 224, 225, 226] The literature often refers to the core as a three-dimensional canister formed by co-activation of the respiratory diaphragm as the roof, transversus abdominis as the sides, and the pelvic floor at the bottom.[227, 228, 229] Together, the bony pelvis and lower core muscles delineate the abdomen. I will refer to this inseparable group of muscles as the lower core muscles, or the traditional core.

Traditional Core

The lower core muscles, PFM, TVA, and RD, or what I call the "traditional core muscles," are inseparable in function. The group of abdominal core muscles formed by co-activation of the respiratory diaphragm, transversus abdominis, and the pelvic floor makes a 3-D "abdominal canister."[230] Activation of all of the muscles in this canister is necessary for "abdominal contents to be controlled and for contraction of transversus abdominis to increase the pressure in the abdominal cavity."[231]

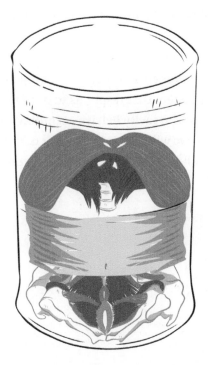

FIGURE 5.7 TRADITIONAL CORE MUSCLES

Intra-abdominal Pressure

What is intra-abdominal pressure, or IAP? It is "defined as the steady-state pressure concealed within the abdominal cavity resulting from the interaction between the abdominal wall and viscera; IAP oscillates according to respiratory phase and abdominal wall resistance."[232] The abdominal cavity is neatly delineated by the lower core muscles and lower portion of the bony core canister. The "roof" of the abdominal cavity is the RD, which is always moving. Therefore, abdominal cavity volume and pressure are in constant flux.

Even when we are physically resting, our body is still breathing, and the volumes of the abdomen and thorax are constantly adjusting to one another. Our respiratory diaphragm is constantly contracting and releasing (15,000–20,000 times per day) to keep us alive. The lower core muscles are consistently responding and adapting to the ever-changing pressures in our rib cage (thorax) and abdomen. The body can't uncouple IAP from trunk muscle co-contraction.[233, 234] In fact, it is impossible to co-contract trunk muscles "without generating IAP and ITP [intra-thoracic pressure], or conversely to generate IAP without trunk muscle co-contraction and increased ITP."[235] In other words, our abdomen and thorax work together as an interdependent pressure system that responds to our breath. The pressure changes in our thoracic cavity behave according to pneumatic (air/gas) physics (which we will look at in Chapter 6, The Breathing Core), and those in our abdominal cavity behave according to hydraulic (fluid) physics.[236]

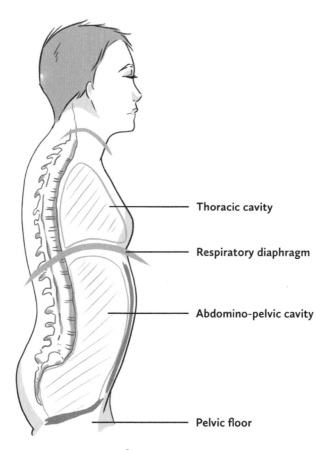

Thoracic cavity

Respiratory diaphragm

Abdomino-pelvic cavity

Pelvic floor

FIGURE 5.8 INTRA-ABDOMINAL PRESSURE

Because the RD is a postural muscle, I often see it being used as a substitute for posture control when another piece of the core is not functioning properly. This substitution adaptation can appear as breath holding, rib flaring, or an increase in the diameter of the abdomen, which I call "poofing out" (as opposed to the dome or "pooch" we talked about when the RA is substituting for another member of the core team).

Therefore, when assessing the lower core muscle function, watch for the TVA to engage inward just prior to or with limb movement. It's subtle. Watch, feel, or listen for breath holding or an *increase* in abdominal or thoracic diameter. When the abdominal muscles appear to be bulging outwardly, or the ribs flare when the respiratory diaphragm becomes rigid, this is the body's way of creating the trunk stability required for limb movement. While this accomplishes the task, it is not sustainable. The inefficient stabilization or trunk rigidity is created by an increase in IAP, which inhibits the TVA from proper recruitment. Once this is recognized, the client or practitioner can be creative and use any movement or activity of daily living to help retrain the PFM and TVA to engage properly prior to moving a limb without holding the breath. Success comes when this movement or activity is meaningful to the client. (More on this in Chapter 7, The Mindful Core.) In the meantime, all of this has to happen while we are breathing: the PFM, TVA, and respiratory diaphragm work together for IAP and trunk stability.

This can be plenty of material for a full rehabilitation plan for someone with low back pain, or as a core program in conjunction with a traditional ankle, knee, or hip program. What about upper quadrant issues? Remember that the intra-*thoracic* pressure is always changing as well, because we are always breathing, and the diaphragm moves to bring air in and out of our lungs all day and all night long. Just as I include the rib basket as part of the bony core, I include the muscles of the thorax as part of the muscular core. I also include certain scapular stabilizing muscles, which I call the "wings," in the sustainable core group.

"Wings"

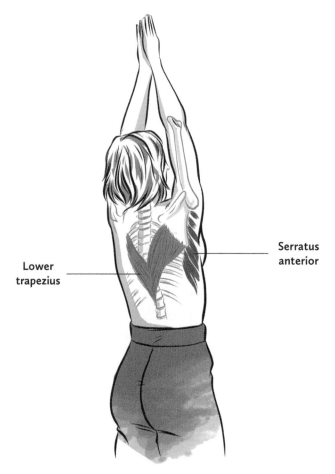

Serratus
anterior

Lower
trapezius

FIGURE 5.9 WINGS

In Latin, the root "*cor*" means heart. The heart lives in the thorax. In my yoga teacher training, my instructor used to say "the wings protect the heart" as she cued our scapular bones away from our ears. In sports medicine and rehabilitation, "winging" of the scapulae (also called *scapula alata*) is a condition where the serratus anterior muscle (SA) and/or the lower trapezius muscle (LT) are not functioning properly. When they are not functioning properly, the medial or lateral border of the scapulae appear to "wing" or fly off the thorax. When there is paralysis of the serratus anterior or trapezius, one cannot raise their arms above the level of the shoulder.[237] When acting alone, the serratus anterior muscle protracts the scapula and the lower trapezius muscle depresses and aids the upper trapezius in upwardly rotating the scapula. When the SA and LT co-contract functionally, they upwardly rotate the shoulder blades.[238]

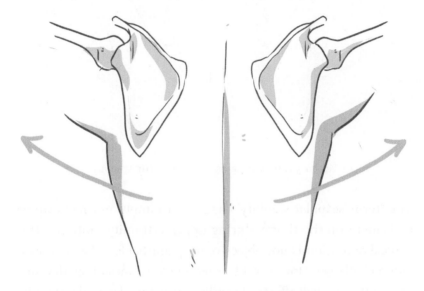

FIGURE 5.10 UPWARD ROTATION OF THE SCAPULA

In orthopedics, the assessment for winging scapulae, or a long thoracic nerve palsy, is the "wall push-up test" where the patient is asked to perform a push-up away from the wall while the practitioner observes for winging of the scapulae.[239] In contrast, downward rotation of the scapulae is accomplished by the latissimus dorsi, levator scapulae, rhomboids, and the pectoralis major and minor muscles co-contracting. When the SA and LT properly co-contract, they connect the scapulae bones to the mid-thorax, that is, they "stabilize" the shoulder blades.

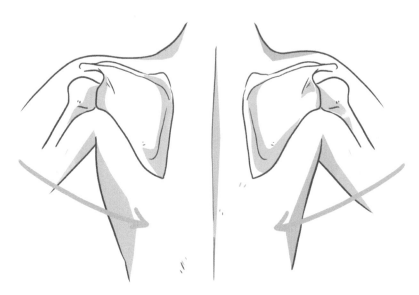

FIGURE 5.11 DOWNWARD ROTATION OF THE SCAPULA

The "term 'scapular stability' has come to imply 'normal' scapula movement on the thorax during upper extremity motions...this clinical definition is not objective or quantifiable,"[240] which presents a challenge. However, I learned in basic kinesiology that one cannot throw a ball effectively without functional scapular stability strength and that scapular stability requires trunk muscle or stability. Research supports the fact that central core muscle stability is necessary, and trunk muscle activation also precedes upper limb movement.[241, 242, 243, 244, 245, 246, 247, 248, 249]

Take a look at the connected anatomy of the serratus anterior muscle with the external oblique muscle (Figure 5.12). Visually, they are continuous and make up the sides of the can in the core cylinder model we are building. They interdigitate and create a basket weave near the axilla (the armpit). Before we move our arm in space, in the shoulder blade—where the "socket" of the shoulder's ball-and-socket joint is located—a team of muscles works together to stabilize the scapula on the thoracic cylinder.

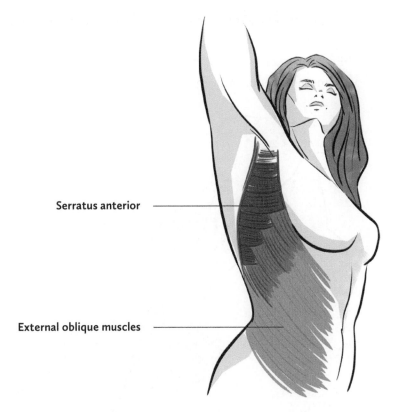

Serratus anterior

External oblique muscles

FIGURE 5.12 THE SERRATUS ANTERIOR AND EXTERNAL OBLIQUE MUSCLE WEAVE

Earlier in my career, the concept of scapular dyskenesis[250, 251, 252] was a popular explanation for rotator cuff impingement in the subacromial space of the shoulder. It was standard practice to use posture training and scapular stabilization strengthening techniques to counteract shoulder pain[253, 254, 255] Even though there is a correlation between breathing pattern disorders and scapular dyskinesis,[256] we know now that there is no evidence to support that poor posture is related to pain.[257] Lewis (2011) suggests that subacromial impingement might be a clinical illusion,[258] and a meta-analysis showed no relationship between acromio-humeral distance and pain.[259] In fact, slouching might even be a protective response.[260] Another study, with 1030 subjects, concludes: "*Psychological* factors were consistently associated with patient-rated outcome, whereas clinical examination findings associated with a specific structural diagnosis were not" (emphasis added).[261] Nonetheless, exploring movement in a safe setting may help. "Progressive exercise training independent from specific scapular stabilization exercises provides decreased disability and pain severity in impingement syndrome."[262]

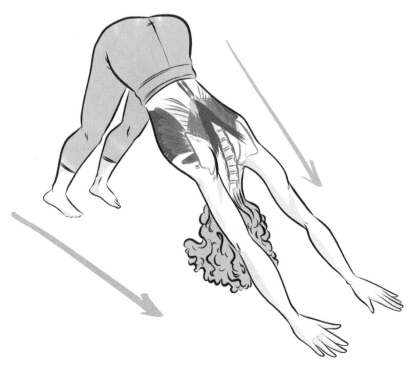

FIGURE 5.13 DOWNWARD-FACING DOG WINGS

In the clinic and on the mat, I look at the coordination of all of the muscles in the trunk, including the scapular stabilizers. Are they functioning together like a team in the desired movement? Is the scapula, and therefore the socket of the arm bone, in an optimal position to co-contract the muscles of the rotator cuff and the entire kinetic chain? McQuade, Borstad, and de Oliveira (2016) note that it's not the balance of the LT and SA that matter.[263] "Rather, all that is required is that the net moment satisfies the Newtonian condition for dynamic equilibrium (from Newton's second law of motion)"[264] for scapular stability, and equal forces are not mandatory. Scapular thoracic (ST) position depends on the task and symphony of coordinated muscles.

The authors note, "it may be more accurate to conceptualize ST function as an energy transfer system rather than an anatomical structural base of support."[265] Furthermore, they recommend looking at muscle coordination patterns and the synergy of the scapulo-thoracic muscles and suggest that "facilitating muscle recruitment with the scapula away from its 'ideal' position may be the most effective."[266]

I agree, and have observed that the scapulae respond best to the next movement task with more resilience and options if they are muscularly set up in position somewhere in the midrange of motion, versus hanging out at end-range on the ligaments and passive soft tissue. The scapulae won't have anywhere to go if they are at end-range elevation, depression, protraction, or retraction. We will explore this in the cat and cow exercise in Chapter 11, Therapeutic Physical-Energetic Practices.

Returning to the core cylinder concept, we need the lower core muscles to provide proximal stability for the scapulae to attach to the trunk to allow for distal mobility of the arm and hand. In throwing sports, such as baseball or javelin, the velocity and force of the object thrown come from the weight transfer in the legs, which translates through the hip and trunk muscles into the arm and the energy release through the fingers of the athlete. The translation of forces within the muscular system is known as the *kinetic chain theory*.[267]

Kinetic Chain Theory

Understanding the kinetic chain theory allows the practitioner to look at the entire system of muscle players when considering the mechanics of the upper extremities.[268, 269, 270, 271, 272, 273, 274] For example, in a tennis stroke, the force to hit the ball comes from the foot contacting the ground, and the ground reactive force travels through the legs, pelvis, torso, scapula, shoulder, elbow, wrist, hand, racket, then ball. In classic "tennis elbow," or lateral epicondylitis, "Although the source of pain may indeed be the lateral elbow, it may be the anatomic 'victim,' but not the 'culprit' of the pathology."[275] The imbalance of load transfer could be from a number of muscle imbalances in this entire chain. In baseball pitchers, decreased lumbo-pelvic stability was correlated with increased elbow vagus stress and shoulder horizontal abduction stress and was correlated to increased upper extremity injury risk.[276]

Another study determined that "Core exercises are likely to enhance trunk stabilization to improve upper extremity function. It is possible for core exercises to be adapted for patients."[277] Trunk exercises helped facilitate skilled motor behavior of the upper extremities. Other research revealed that "greater shoulder dysfunction was correlated with higher balance and stability deficiency."[278] The authors suggest that "therapists and trainers should consider incorporating balance training as an integral component of core stability into rehabilitation of athletes with shoulder dysfunction."[279] Again, when assessing the upper core muscle function, I look at how the entire core canister is working to support a moving limb; it doesn't matter whether the moving limb is the upper or lower extremity. If the most unstable part of the system is the connection of the upper extremity to the trunk at the scapula, exercises to restore scapular muscle balance have been shown to increase strength in adjacent joints.[280, 281]

Remember that the SA protracts the scapulae, and the test for a weak SA is the "wall push-up." When our hands are on the ground, we close the kinetic chain and reverse the proximal and distal moving joints/parts. Exercises where the distal end of a limb are fixed are termed "closed-chain exercises." Conversely, exercises where the hands or feet are freely moving in space are called "open-chain exercises." In upper extremity, closed-chain exercises, such as planks, push-ups, or downward-facing dog pose, coordinated SA function is important. If winging or lack of SA/LT coordination is present, we can modify the assessment (a closed-chain exercise) and turn it into a rehabilitation exercise. This is supported in the literature; the "standard push-up plus with ipsilateral—same side—leg extension" (SPP-ILE) exercise "may be a useful exercise for subjects with scapular winging."[282] A "push-up plus" is the name for the action of protraction of the scapula beyond neutral in a standard push-up (on the knees or toes). In the above study, the authors propose that the pectoralis major (PM) muscle is recruited to compensate, or assist, a weak serratus anterior (SA) to protract the scapula. I see this on the mat often, and will discuss common substitutions in the coming pages. Just as coordinated activity of the deep abdominal muscles and the wings are important in closed-chain activities, they are important to consider with open-chain activities as well.

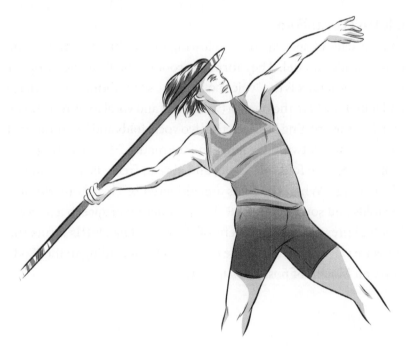

FIGURE 5.14 JAVELIN

When assessing sports function, again, we need to look at how the entire kinetic chain is functioning in a given task. Let's further consider the biomechanics of a ball or javelin throw, an upper extremity open-chain activity. The ground reaction force and the speed, angle, and height of the release are all factors, and muscle force and coordination are needed at all the joint angles—from the feet to the hands. In order for the ground reaction force to translate through the body to the object being thrown, we need central stability, or core strength, for the distal mobility and torque to translate to distance and speed of the object being thrown. The foot hits the ground, and the PFM, TVA, RD, and scapular stabilizers translate the force through the arm. Often, an athlete will add a vocalization, like a grunt or shout, at the release of a javelin or shot put. Why? It turns out that the vocal folds, or the muscles of speech and swallowing, also play a role in pressure management and core stability.

Glottis/Vocal Folds

The muscles of speech and swallowing in the throat complete the core cylinder model. They form the roof of the thoracic or upper core.[283] The larynx is the "voice box," or the space formed by cartilage and muscles where the trachea (wind pipe) and vocal folds reside. The glottis is the opening between the two vocal folds and "is considered to be the valve between the lungs and the mouth."[284] When the glottis is abducted, the folds are open, and air can freely flow in and out of the lungs. When the folds are adducted or closed, air vibrates the folds and sound is created. The production of speech and voice involves pressure management of the core. The glottis forms the pressure valve at the top of the core cylinder according to the "Soda Pop Can Model" of postural support.[285]

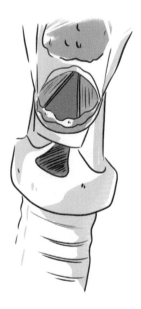 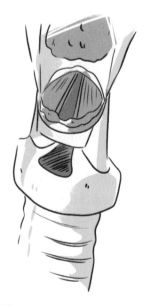

FIGURE 5.15 THE GLOTTIS

Mary Massery is a physical therapist who works with children with cystic fibrosis, a condition that affects the elasticity of the lungs, where mechanical breathing support is often necessary in the form of a tracheostomy. Massery noticed that if a tracheostomy valve wasn't sealed or fitting correctly in the throat, the children couldn't create enough *intra-abdominal pressure for postural control*. They were over-recruiting their accessory breathing muscles for posture instead of breathing. She proposed that the RD was the primary pressure regulator and that global, interconnected postural trunk control comes from the top of the can (vocal folds), through the center of the can (diaphragm), to the bottom of the can (pelvic floor).[286] Again, breathing is correlated with the pelvic floor,[287] and there is a continuous fascial connection from the pelvic floor through the RD to the vocal folds.[288] "Pelvic floor physical therapists have long utilized breathing cues with exercises, and are now starting to incorporate vocalization tasks."[289] Massery noted that everyday activities like pushing doors, giving a little extra push during a bowel movement, or lifting a toddler into a car often involved glottal strategies.[290] Currently, there are several emerging continuing education courses for physical therapists that discuss the research and clinical correlations of the glottis with the rest of the core.[291, 292, 293, 294]

Three Diaphragm Muscles

The physical therapy school I attended was housed in an osteopathic school. I learned that "Working on the diaphragm muscle and the connected diaphragms is part of the respiratory-circulatory osteopathic model."[295] The materials I studied included *five* diaphragms (tentorium cerebelli, tongue, thoracic outlet, thoracic diaphragm, and pelvic floor) in their assessments of core function. I focus on three diaphragms: the pelvic floor, thoracic/respiratory diaphragm, and vocal folds. The function and coordination of the diaphragms cannot be dissected apart. In performing arts medicine rehabilitation, a study showed that "Activation of the PFMs during singing improved PFM strength."[296]

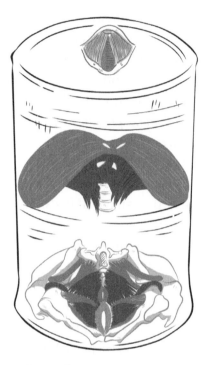

FIGURE 5.16 THE THREE DIAPHRAGMS

In 2011, Matthew Taylor, a PT and founding yoga therapist, described "a model for patients to understand the systems relationships of health and how they can create a new way toward comfort and quality of life by understanding their 3 diaphragms."[297] In an updated YouTube video from 2015,[298] Taylor simplifies the anatomy of the three diaphragms and introduces the interconnectedness of the three diaphragms, the nervous system, and stress. Spoiler alert: the vagus nerve plays a huge role in the communication between the three diaphragms and our central nervous system. And, in yoga, the three diaphragms are interconnected through an advanced "energetic-locking" or binding practice called "engaging the *bandhas*." We will discuss this locking practice more in Chapter 8, The Energetic Core. For now, I want to bring your attention to the interconnectedness of the traditional core and the three diaphragm muscles. When the pelvis, rib basket, and head are stacked on a neutral spine, the three diaphragm muscles become parallel, and when the sustainable core muscles are engaged, a unique action emerges: axial extension, or axial elongation.

Axial Extension and Co-contraction

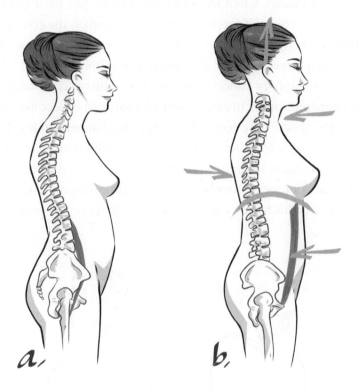

FIGURE 5.17 AXIAL EXTENSION

Traditionally, the trunk and spine move in four directions: flexion, extension, rotation, and side-bending. The fifth spinal movement, axial extension, "is defined as a simultaneous reduction of both the primary and secondary curves of the spine."[299] Recall that the primary curve of the spine is kyphosis, and secondary curves are the cervical and lumbar lordotic curves. When all three curves reduce, the length of the entire spine increases. According to yoga instructor and author Leslie Kaminoff, axial extension requires neutral alignment, and it involves a shift in the tone and orientation of the three diaphragms. As rehabilitation professionals, we might be interested in how the body lengthens the spine, because this action decompresses the vertebrae and helps reduce lumbar and disc loads (see Figure 4.8).

I believe that axial extension is the same movement seen in dance and Pilates, when students are cued to "lift their crowns." Joseph Pilates himself promoted exercises based on the concepts of a balanced body and mind, and drew from the approach espoused by the early Greeks.[300] He called his system "Contrology."[301] I think Pilates' Contrology concept taps into the elusive co-contraction and coordination of muscles around a joint that decompress or widen the spaces between joints. When this happens in the trunk, the entire spine lengthens through the coordinated action of the three diaphragms. I believe it is related and bound to the body–mind connection due to the coordination of the three diaphragms and the implications this has on our breathing efficiency and posture.

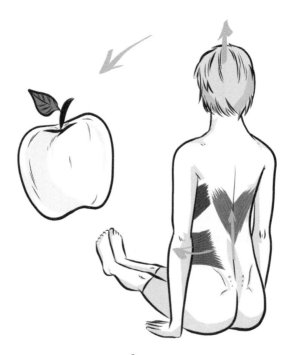

FIGURE 5.18 COORDINATION

Exploring the Sustainable Core Muscles in Seated Axial Extension

Building on the understanding that a neutral spine zone creates the best length–tension relationship for the sustainable core muscles (particularly, the three diaphragms), and for initially finding axial extension, I often have clients explore relaxation and contraction of these muscles in neutral spine. I invite you to explore your sustainable core muscles in a seated position with me:

- Sit on the edge of a firm chair or other surface with your feet on the ground.
- Find a neutral pelvis, thorax, and head position (see Chapter 4 for more details).
- What happens if you attempt to "lift your crown" or "float" your head like a balloon toward the sky?
- For some people, lifting the crown in this position requires a lot of effort. If this is your experience, pause here and continue breathing. See if you can maintain that axial extension for 3–6 more steady breaths.
- If axial extension is achievable for you and your breathing is steady, try adding further exploration:
  - Can you relax the *pelvic floor muscles* on the inhalation and lightly contract them on your exhalation? (See the instructions in Chapter 11 for the reverse Kegel for more detail.) Are you maintaining axial extension throughout the exercise?
  - Are you able to engage your *transverse abdominis (TVA) muscle* on the exhalation and relax it on the inhalation? Are you maintaining axial extension throughout the exercise? Note that this requires a long, soft, slow, complete exhalation to perform correctly.
  - If you are able to relax and contract your TVA with the breath, now try shifting the amount of release of the TVA during the inhalation. On the exhale, contract the TVA as before (perhaps to about 40–60% of maximal contraction), then release the TVA about 10 percent during the

inhalation (consciously relaxing and lengthening the TVA on the inhalation, but not all the way). Continue breathing while contracting and relaxing the TVA in this midrange of motion. Exhale and contract, inhale and relax, for another 6–10 breath cycles.

- Check your shoulder blade position. If your scapulae are protracted, use your "wings" to slightly retract them to a more neutral position and continue to maintain axial extension.

• Finally, are you able to contract and relax your PFM *and* your TVA muscles with your inhale *and* exhale while maintaining axial extension?
  - Explore the ranges of motion of the PFM and TVA with the breath, without changing your bony core position.

Ask yourself: Can you make your neck longer? What happens if you become aware of your diaphragms and breath? Can you breathe freely and maintain axial extension? To do this requires a lot of teamwork from the core muscles, and I tend to see three main trends in people who are *unable* to maintain a sustainable core muscle symphony:

• chronic passive end-range postures
• unmanaged intra-abdominal pressure
• persistent pain or chronic psychological stress.

Barriers to Sustainable Core Recruitment

Barrier 1: *Chronic Poor Posture with Crossed Syndromes*

Earlier in my career, I relied on the research that poor posture leads to poor breathing patterns,[302] and that faulty breathing patterns are statistically correlated with neck pain.[303] From a purely mechanistic lens, this still holds true, but we can't reduce the problem to a simple alignment issue. This hypothesis is supported by Vladimir Janda's theory on upper- and lower-crossed syndromes.[304, 305] Janda's muscle imbalance syndrome premise is that "as certain muscle groups differentiate into tonic dominance or phasic dominance, they develop the tendency to either shorten or tighten (tonic dominance) or to lengthen or weaken (phasic dominance)."[306]

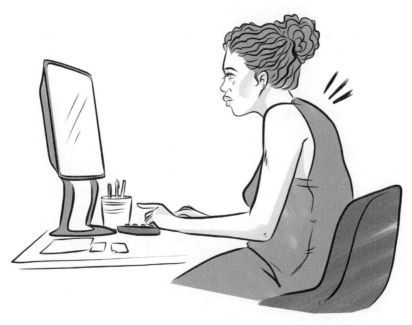

FIGURE 5.19 POOR POSTURE

Upper-crossed syndrome (UCS), also referred to as proximal or shoulder girdle crossed syndrome, is characterized by *facilitation* (chronic overactivation) of the upper trapezius, levator scapula, sternocleidomastoid, and pectoralis muscles, as well as *inhibition* of the deep cervical flexors, lower trapezius, and serratus anterior.[307] This can lead to specific postural changes in UCS, "including forward head posture, increased cervical lordosis and thoracic kyphosis, elevated and protracted shoulders, and rotation or abduction and winging of the scapulae."[308]

Forward head posture is associated with breathing pattern disorders,[309] decreased mobility of the lower rib cage,[310] shortening and weakening of the accessory breathing muscles,[311] has immediate effects on the respiratory function,[312] and produces reduced vital capacity even in healthy adults.[313]

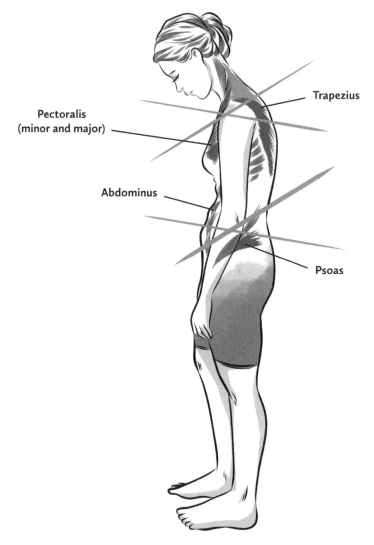

Pectoralis
(minor and major)

Trapezius

Abdominus

Psoas

FIGURE 5.20 CROSS SYNDROMES

Lower-crossed syndrome (LCS) is characterized by *facilitation* of the thoraco-lumbar extensors, rectus femoris, and iliopsoas, as well as *inhibition* of the abdominals (particularly transversus abdominis) and the gluteal muscles.[314] Lower-crossed syndrome is sometimes also called pelvic-crossed syndrome, and a combination of UCS and LCS is called *layered* syndrome.[315] The lower-crossed "imbalance results in an anterior tilt of the pelvis, increased flexion of the hips, and a compensatory hyper-lordosis in the lumbar spine."[316] Upper, lower, and pelvic-crossed syndromes consider the mechanics of the muscles in the sagittal plane. Wallden (2014) also proposes a common pattern in the transverse plane muscles, called "middle-crossed syndrome," which involves the reciprocal inhibition of the arm swing during walking.[317]

I often observe these same crossed muscle patterns of overactive and underactive muscles in the studio, especially in those who lead a sedentary lifestyle and primarily sit for work or hobbies. On the other end of the spectrum, people who specialize or train in one endurance sport, like ultra-marathon runners, also exhibit these patterns. Josephine Key sees this in the clinic and has discussed the implications these postures and muscle imbalances have on IAP.[318, 319] These patterns are observed clinically with an overuse of extrinsic or superficial core muscles and deficient intrinsic control of the traditional core muscles. The pressure regulation is disturbed because the shape of the thoracic and abdominal cavities is changed, the RD's function is compromised, and "The IAP generated provides suboptimal support for breathing and postural control."[320]

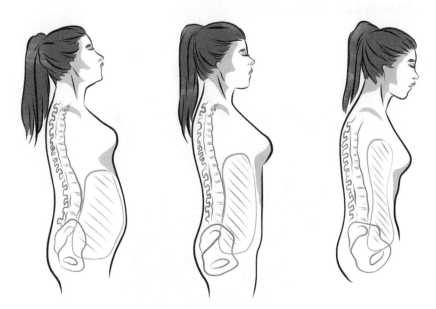

FIGURE 5.21 PELVIC CROSS SYNDROME AND IAP

Barrier 2: *Unmanaged Intra-abdominal Pressure*

The relationship between intra-abdominal pressure and spinal stability is a central component to a sustainable core. Research reveals that intra-abdominal pressure (IAP) "contributes, at least in part, to spinal stability,"[321] and is "an important mechanism in central component to postural trunk stabilisation and control."[322] We normally generate increased IAP in response to jumping and sudden trunk-loading tasks.[323] "It is suggested that it is not necessarily the absolute trunk load which governs the level of IAP but more the relative effort of the task."[324] There is a difference between healthy IAP and strain. Coordination of all three diaphragms with the TVA are needed to move air *up* through the glottis, like during a cough[325] or speaking. And they also work together to move air, liquid, and food *downward*, to swallow,[326] urinate,[327] and defecate.[328] Normal defecation does not involve straining, and the combination of forces needed for a normal bowel movement is traditionally called a Valsalva maneuver (VM). The VM "often is defined as 15 seconds of expiration with an *open glottis* against 40mmHg pressure" (emphasis added).[329] In a normal Valsalva maneuver, the RD and PFM move cranially (toward the head) and the abdominal muscles contract.[330]

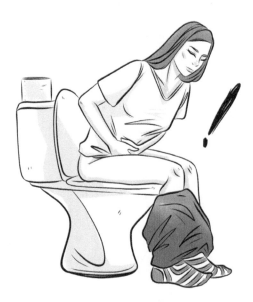

FIGURE 5.22 TOILET

"Valsalva and straining are different tasks with different PFM acti-vation patterns."[331] During *straining*, the glottis *closes*, the RD stays in the *inspiration* position (cranially), and the PFM move *caudally* (downward). When the pelvic floor moves downward or caudally, the neck of the bladder lengthens with it. "An adequate pelvic floor muscle contraction (PFMC) elevates the bladder neck (BN) and sta-bilizes it during increased intra-abdominal pressure (IAP),"[332] main-taining adequate closure for continence. The PFM are stiffer with Valsalva resulting in better bladder neck support whereas *straining* leads to more PFM and bladder neck descent.[333] One preliminary investigation explored the changes in bladder shape distortion as a proxy for pelvic floor muscle displacement during respiratory and phonatory tasks. It concluded, "When cuing pelvic floor to contract, healthy individuals showed shortening of bladder length and most lengthened during strain."[334]

Even with an open glottis, the Valsalva maneuver affects our heart rate and blood pressure.[335] In a normal VM, this healthy "push" is accompanied by an increase in intra-*thoracic* pressure and followed by vagus nerve inhibition and sympathetic nervous system stim-ulation.[336] Problems may arise when there is chronic straining or overused muscle substitutions. One study noted, "Possible harmful effects of high intra-abdominal pressure on the pelvic girdle," and concluded that "the size of the load induced by IAP on the pelvic girdle seems to be sufficient to cause pain in patients with PGP (pelvic girdle pain)," and that "It seems worthwhile to give patients with PGP instructions to reduce IAP as much as possible during activities."[337]

In other words, in a normal bowel movement, the PFM, TVA, and RD work together, without straining or closing the glottis. This implies a "submaximal" (midrange, not tightened to full end-range) contraction of the PFM. During straining, however, the glottis is closed, and the PFM descend. The terms "strain" and "Valsalva maneuver" should not be used interchangeably, one study cautions. It adds that patients "have to be instructed carefully to allow appro-priate interpretation of data."[338] "A maximal [PFM contraction] may increase the IAP and thereby prevent BN elevation."[339] Why is this an issue? It's not an issue in itself, as this muscle coordination exists because sometimes a little push is necessary to get the job done. It's okay to occasionally strain or lengthen the pelvic floor. In fact, this needs to happen to birth a baby vaginally. Problems occur when the tissue is chronically and repeatedly stretched to end-range, or is acutely lengthened beyond its maximal stretch capacity (ruptured).

Coordination of the PFM, TVA, and RD, and constant adjustments in intra-abdominal pressure, are needed for maintaining an upright posture.[340, 341, 342, 343] "The IAP mechanism for stabilizing the lumbar spine appears preferable in tasks that demand trunk extensor movement such as lifting or jumping. This mechanism can increase spine stability without the additional co-activation of erector spinae muscles."[344] In fact, research determined that highest intra-abdominal pressures in healthy patients "are generated during coughing and jumping...and patients with higher [body mass index] and chronic cough appear to generate significant elevation in IAP."[345] A prolonged or sudden increase in IAP "has been considered responsible for adverse effects in trauma and other abdominal catastrophes as well as in formation and recurrence of hernias."[346] In other words, if we close the glottis, increase our IAP and ITP, and bear down long enough without breathing, non-resilient and fragile tissue might strain.

Clinically, I see a correlation between poor sustainable core muscle management and poor trunk pressure management in most hernia, diastasis recti, prolapse, and intervertebral disc issues. Teaching breathing coordinated with high-load activities is key in helping these clients recover. Research bears this out. Athletic rehabilitation for core stability is not achieved by just strengthening the core muscles in isolation, but by coordination of muscles utilizing IAP regulation.[347] I have noticed that when clients and athletes are not managing their IAP while moving, they are often not breathing efficiently either.

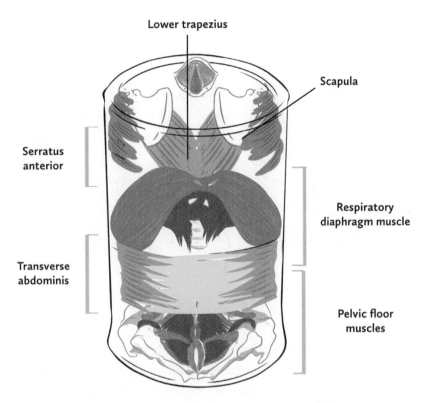

Lower trapezius

Scapula

Serratus anterior

Respiratory diaphragm muscle

Transverse abdominis

Pelvic floor muscles

FIGURE 5.23 THE ABDOMINAL AND THORAX CANISTER

Barrier 3: *Persistent Overuse of Accessory Breathing Muscles*
As a licensed manual therapist, I have had the unique opportunity of palpating the quality of soft tissue in clients. I was trained in Active Release Techniques®, or ART, which is a soft tissue treatment method that focuses on relieving tissue tension via the removal of fibrosis or adhesions that develop in tissue that is overloaded with repetitive use.[348, 349] Strikingly, a high number of clients have overactive and/or fibrotic *accessory* breathing muscles (the group of muscles used for breathing beyond the respiratory diaphragm muscle).

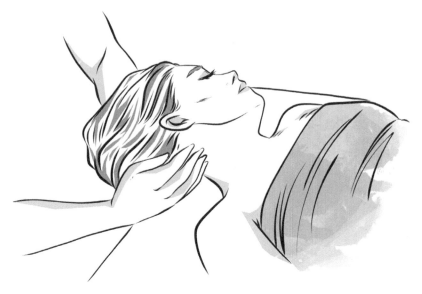

FIGURE 5.24 NECK MASSAGE

The common factor in all three of these barriers to a sustainable core is that there is presence of a breathing pattern disorder (BPD). Did the BPD or the core muscle imbalance come first? It doesn't matter, as we can't separate the functions of posture, breathing, and pressure management in the core. The RD will continue to breathe for us. Recall that every muscle of the trunk is both a respiratory and a postural muscle, especially the diaphragm. Posture management includes IAP management. Massery discovered that "When the patient has lost the ability to generate, regulate, and/or maintain appropriate internal pressures in both the thoracic and abdominal chambers, the mechanics of breathing, as well as numerous other body functions, may be impaired."[350] When the RD is pulling the double duties of breathing *and* postural stabilization, the body recruits the help of accessory breathing muscles to get enough air exchange. This strategy works fine in the short term, but it is not sustainable. Ideally, the PF, TVA, and wings are working together (co-contracting at midrange in relation to the load of the task) for postural support while allowing the RD and glottis to breathe and speak. In other words, if the RD is not available for breathing while it is being used as a postural stability muscle, other muscles are recruited to breathe, and the symphony of core muscles is not balanced. This is a breathing pattern disorder in itself. Before we discuss breathing pattern disorders, let's discuss normal breathing patterns.

6

THE BREATHING CORE

Efficient breathing is the key to a sustainable core. Inefficient breathing could result in muscular imbalance, motor control alterations, and physiological adaptations that are capable of modifying movement.[1] Thankfully, mindful breathing and meditation can help decrease stress and related muscle tension.[2, 3] Recall from the previous chapter that the respiratory diaphragm muscle (RD) is the most fatigue-resistant muscle in the body,[4] and that "except in cases of paralysis, the diaphragm is always used for breathing. The issue is whether it is being used efficiently or not."[5]

What exactly is efficient use of the diaphragm? Although the diaphragm is the main inspiratory muscle, expanding the chest wall during breathing is an integrated process that involves many muscles, in particular the internal and external intercostal muscles. "Three main sets of muscles are active when you breathe normally: the *intercostal muscles*, the *abdominal muscles*, and the *respiratory diaphragm*."[6] The volume of air moved into or out of the lungs during a normal breath is called the tidal volume (TV). If we were to graph it, the normal inhalation and exhalation makes a tide or sine wave, shown in the middle of Figure 6.1 as TV.

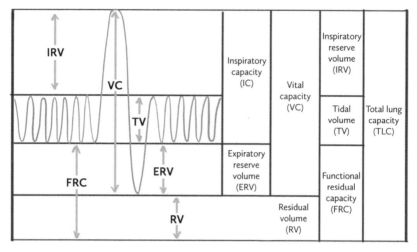

FIGURE 6.1 TIDAL VOLUME

In quiet, normal breathing, the RD only requires energy to contract for *inhaling*. Quiet *exhalation* does not require any active muscle contractions; the lungs expel the tidal volume with passive recoil of the domes of the diaphragm. When our body requires more oxygen, beyond quiet breathing (for example, during exercise), our thorax and lungs have room for extra intake. This extra inhalation capacity volume is called *inspiratory reserve volume* (IRV). In contrast, when we need an extra push, the muscles in the abdomen contract and we can expel air below our tidal volume. This maximum exhalation volume is called *expiratory reserve* (ERV).

Together, our tidal volume plus our inspiratory and expiratory reserve volumes (TV + IRV + ERV) equals our *vital capacity* (VC). The vital capacity is the total amount of air we can voluntarily move in and out of our lungs. We also have a residual volume (RV), or the air that remains in our lungs after a complete forced expiration. The residual volume functions to keep the alveoli open even after maximum expiration.[7] When we get the "wind knocked out of us," like in a blow to the solar plexus in sports, it is our ERV that is passively expelled, and our RV that keeps our lungs inflated, still allowing oxygen exchange while we "catch our breath" and recover. Expiratory reserve volume plus this residual volume equals the functional residual capacity (FRC). I am interested in the muscles that activate to bring in this extra inspiratory volume, and the ones that contract to expel the expiratory reserve volume. These are the accessory inspiration and accessory expiration muscles. Let's continue to discuss normal breathing, then see how these accessory muscles interact and interfere with cultivating a sustainable core.

Breathing Mechanics
Inspiration

In quiet breathing, the respiratory diaphragm contracts and performs about 70–80 percent of the work for inhalation.[8] "Inhalations can take place only as a result of muscular activity,"[9] while exhalation can be passive. The intercostals and scalenes assist in picking up the remaining 20–30 percent.[10, 11] "Minor activity of the scalenes occurs with even a light breath, but more obvious visual and palpable activity occurs when demand is increased."[12]

During inspiration, the diaphragm actively contracts, flattens, and descends while the lower ribs expand. The caudal descent of the RD displaces the abdominal and pelvic organs (intestines, bladder, and uterus, if present) downward. This increases IAP and creates outward motion or distension of the anterior abdominal wall and downward pressure on the PFM.[13]

The pelvic floor and respiratory diaphragm muscles are functionally parallel to each other. Together, they move together synchronistically like a piston engine during quiet breathing. Continuing an inhalation beyond the tidal volume, the *abdominal* muscles can stay relaxed and passively expand, or they can resist the expansion and *eccentrically* contract.[14]

INHALE **EXHALE**

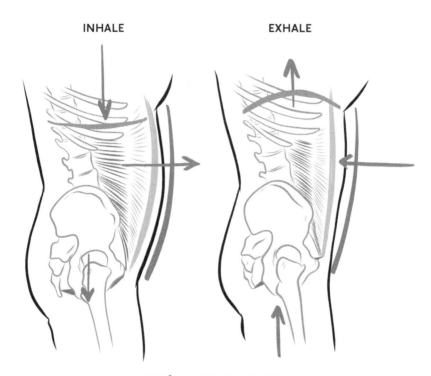

FIGURE 6.2 STANDING REVERSE KEGEL

"Breathing requires synchronized concentric activity of the diaphragm and pelvic floor, as well as eccentric activity of all muscles that insert into the thorax and abdominal wall muscles."[15] Altered trunk muscle sequencing during breathing can alter motor control patterns of the core muscles, resulting in pain and/or dysfunction.[16]

Mary Massery reminds us that breathing is "influenced by gravity in all planes of motion...[and it] is an integral part of multi-system interactions and consequences that simultaneously support respiration and postural control for all motor tasks."[17] Leslie Kaminoff offers "an expanded definition of breathing: '...the taking in and expelling of air in the lungs, caused by changing the shape of the thoracic and abdominal cavities.'" He further notes that "Gravity, posture, activity, habit, and intention...affect the shape-changing activities of the body cavities (breathing)" and that there is individual variety.[18] All these factors will come into play shortly when we consider which breathing exercises to practice.

Accessory Inspiration Muscles

The accessory inspiration muscles play an important role in breathing. They are recruited to lift the thorax when extra inhalation is needed during activity. They include the scalenes, sternocleidomastoid (SCM), upper trapezius (UT),[19] pectoralis major and minor, serratus anterior (SA), latissimus dorsi (LT),[20] iliocostalis thoracis, omohyoid, and subclavius muscles.[21] "The scalenes and accessory muscles including the SCM and upper trapezius musculature are activated normally upon high levels of ventilatory demand or at high lung volumes such as in hyperinflation."[22]

> Although the pectoralis major, pectoralis minor, latissimus dorsi, serratus anterior, and trapezius are not typically considered accessory respiratory muscles, they assume a more respiratory than postural function in the dysfunctional or paradoxical breather and contribute to the faulty pattern of lifting the ribcage up during inspiration.[23]

The accessory inspiration muscles all assist the ribs or clavicles in *elevation* when a deeper breath is needed.[24] They become taxed easily when they are over-recruited, performing the duties of both posture and breathing.

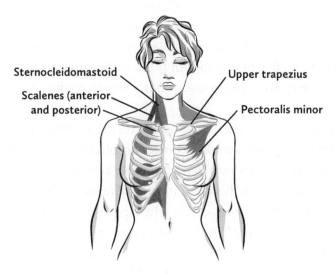

FIGURE 6.3 ACCESSORY INSPIRATION MUSCLES

In patients with diaphragm dysfunction, the accessory respiratory muscles (scalenes and SCM) lift the rib cage to facilitate lung filling during inspiration. These secondary muscles are often tight and hyperactive in patients with chronic neck pain due to deep neck flexor weakness... In faulty respiration patterns, these tight muscles are readily activated and continue to facilitate the patterns of muscle imbalance with each breath.[25]

One type of insufficient chest breathing "occurs when the diaphragm is weak or paralyzed, while the upper accessory muscles are still intact...the accessory muscles are not designed to meet the needs of long-term independent ventilation and are more likely to fatigue and cause respiratory distress."[26] Another study demonstrated that *inspiratory muscle fatigue* (IMF) is correlated with "a rigid proprioceptive postural control strategy, rather than the normal 'multi-segmental' control, which is similar to people with LBP."[27] I see this in the clinic often as well. It is very common for a client who complains of back or neck pain to also exhibit a faulty breathing pattern called "chest breathing," where their sternum rises vertically during inspiration instead of remaining still at rest. Chest breathing is the "most common fault in respiration" and "occurs due to bilateral overactivity in the scalene trapezius, and elevator scapulae musculature."[28] Indeed, these clients typically also complain of tight or sore scalene, upper trapezius, and levator scapulae muscles and, upon palpation, these muscles feel hypertonic and/or fibrotic. Over-recruitment of the accessory breathing muscles has a negative effect on exercise capacity.[29]

While it is detrimental to rely solely on the accessory inspiration muscles throughout our day, resisted inspiratory muscle training (IMT) is beneficial for overall performance and can "have a positive effect on core muscle function independent of specific core training."[30] IMT "elicits resistance to the development of inspiratory muscles fatigue during high-intensity exercise."[31] Inspiratory muscle training improves shuttle run performance in healthy subjects, and "these improvements result in reduced levels of breathlessness, and increase in predicted VO2 max and a perceived improvement in sports performance."[32] In a 2016 study by Tong et al., they showed that functional inspiratory and core muscle training enhances running performance and economy.[33]

Expiration and Accessory Expiration Muscles

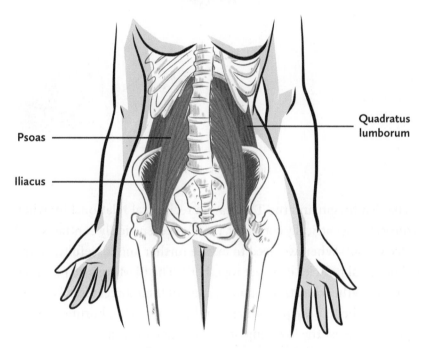

Psoas

Iliacus

Quadratus lumborum

FIGURE 6.4 ACCESSORY EXPIRATION MUSCLES

Normal, quiet, exhalation is accomplished by passive recoil of the respiratory diaphragm muscle back to its resting domed shape when the inspiratory muscles are at rest.[34] Toward the end of a quiet exhalation, the abdominal muscles concentrically contract, the viscera get compressed, and the respiratory diaphragm eccentrically contracts, to prepare to inhale again.

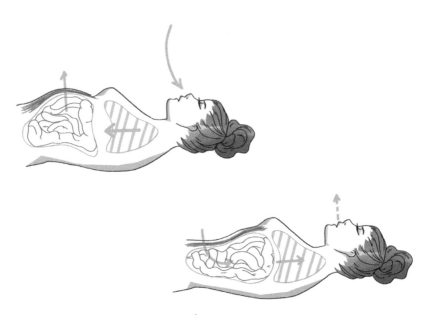

FIGURE 6.5 BELLY BREATH

The diaphragm and the TVA have a reciprocal relationship: when the RD concentrically contracts, the TVA eccentrically contracts, and vice versa.[35] When we need to exhale further and forcefully, all the abdominal muscles contract together.[36] The PFM are also recruited with forceful exhalation,[37] and because of their direct fascial attachment to the RD, the psoas major and quadratus lumborum muscles probably assist the lowering of the ribs and diaphragm.[38]

In the studio, I also see a pattern of overactive and fibrotic accessory expiration muscles—particularly the iliopsoas and quadratus lumborum—in people with chronic stress or faulty breathing. It's possible that the iliopsoas can take over as an accessory breathing muscle if the spine and sacrum are immobile, disturbing the normal functioning of the crura of the diaphragm. The psoas plays an important role in the flight/fight/freeze response.[39, 40, 41, 42, 43, 44] In particular, the iliopsoas muscle contracts in response to life-threatening situations.[45] In my clinical experience, the accessory inhalation and exhalation muscles tend to be hypertonic and/or fibrotic upon palpation in people who report being under extremely stressful or traumatic times in their life. I am inclined to call them "the emergency core" muscles, and will discuss them in the upcoming section Emergency Core Muscles (Accessory Breathing Muscles).

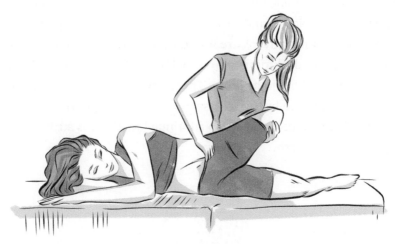

FIGURE 6.6 PSOAS RELEASE

Breathing Pattern Disorders

Chest Breathing

Again, in my experience, breathing pattern disorders (BPD) are typically present in clients who demonstrate uncoordinated core muscle recruitment. "Breathing pattern disorders (BPDs), historically known as hyperventilation syndrome, are being increasingly recognized as an entity of their own."[46] "Breathing Pattern Disorders (BPD)...are abnormal respiratory patterns, specifically related to over-breathing. They range from simple upper chest breathing to, at the end of the scale, hyperventilation."[47] Kaminoff (2006) notes "that hyperventilation refers to the chemical condition of the blood, not to a particular pattern of rapid or shallow breathing."[48] In other words, "Expiration is faulty when the breath is held and not fully exhaled, rib motion is reduced, or paradoxical breathing occurs."[49] *Paradoxical breathing* occurs when "the chest wall moves in on inspiration and out on expiration, in reverse of the normal movements. It may be seen in children with respiratory distress of any cause, which leads to indrawing of the intercostal spaces during inspiration."[50] Paradoxical breathing is not the same as the stress/chest breath discussed in this chapter, and is actually a sign of medical distress. In chest breathing, *the accessory breathing muscles are chronically overused.* Clinically, this appears as overactive and/or fibrotic accessory breathing muscles. Faulty breathing patterns are found in individuals with poor posture,[51] scapular dyskinesis,[52] low back pain[53, 54] neck pain,[55, 56] and temporomandibular joint pain.[57] The faulty thoracic/chest breathing pattern is produced by the accessory muscles of inspiration.[58, 59] The automatic drive for our body to continue breathing is strong, even up to our last breath.

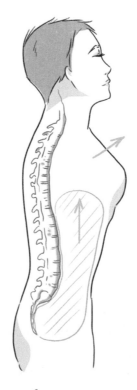

FIGURE 6.7 CHEST BREATHING

The most profound experience I have had of seeing someone use their accessory breathing muscles instead of their sustainable breathing muscles was in my mother-in-law, as she lay on her death bed. I am extremely grateful and fortunate that I was able to witness my husband's mother's final breath on this earth. Her hospice team compassionately educated us on what to expect, and I learned that she would be near the end of her time here when she exhibited a "fish out of water" type of breath. Beth Cavenaugh's thoughtful, educational end-of-life blog describes this phenomenon: "They may appear as though they are opening and closing their mouth without actually breathing. They may have a gasping quality to their breath, known as agonal breathing. Or, their lips will 'puff' out with barely a breath."[60] I was grateful to have had this knowledge in that sacred moment. When the time came, indeed, her breathing shifted and her accessory breathing muscles—specifically her scalenes and sternocleidomastoid—contracted a few last times, almost like gills of a fish opening and closing. Even though her spirit had left her body, her mouth still gaped. It was as if the body had not yet received the signal that it was okay to stop breathing. Instead of panicking, we were able to hold space, witness, and honor her last breaths.

While this was an extreme example at the end of a life, BPD impact day-to-day experience as well. BPD "may cause or contribute to a variety of general health and musculoskeletal conditions (e.g. inappropriate motor control patterns and/or compromised trunk stability). An optimal breathing pattern is typically defined as a three-dimensional abdominal breath resulting in expansion of the lower ribs and has been suggested as an essential component for maintenance of allostasis, posture, and spinal stability."[61] Hyperventilation is also a concern. It may "disrupt mechanisms mediating vestibular compensation [balance]."[62]

In the case of *inspiratory muscle fatigue*, proprioceptive input from the lower back becomes less reliable, disturbing sensory integration and thereby balance.[63] Overall, it appears that BPD/hyperventilation affects the interoceptive sensory and motor systems of the postural control mechanism. Help is available, however, through various therapies and clinical approaches:

Restoring proper breathing mechanics and neuromuscular motor control patterns during breathing may result in a decrease in pain, improved patient outcomes, and overall patient wellbeing associated with their primary musculoskeletal complaint. A comprehensive evaluation of breathing patterns, as a part of an orthopedic examination, may guide a clinician in providing effective and appropriate treatments to decrease pain and improve function.[64]

Anderson and Bliven (2017) found that "grade B evidence exists to support the use of breathing exercises in the treatment of chronic, nonspecific low back pain."[65] There is significant literature available on the impact of BPD on low back, pelvis, SI, and overuse injuries, as well as general pain patterns.[66, 67, 68, 69, 70, 71, 72] Hodges and Moseley (2003) argue that, "at least in some cases, pain may cause the changes in control."[73] "Inefficient breathing could result in muscular imbalance, motor control alterations, and physiological adaptations that are capable of modifying movement"[74] (see Figure 6.7).

Mouth Breathing and Sleep Apnea

Chronic mouth breathing dries out our mucous membranes and comes with a slew of health issues.[75] Mouth breathing is related to *forward head posture*[76, 77, 78, 79] and other suboptimal postural adaptations.[80, 81] Forward head posture and mouth breathing are also related to increased accessory muscle recruitment[82, 83] and have a negative effect on exercise capacity.[84] Mouth breathing compromises adherence to nasal *continuous positive airway pressure* (CPAP) therapy.[85]

CPAP therapy is prescribed for patients with sleep apnea. "Sleep apnea is a potentially serious sleep disorder in which breathing repeatedly stops and starts."[86] Snoring loudly and feeling tired even after a full night's sleep are common indications. Sleep apnea is "a chronic disease that increases the risk of high blood pressure, heart disease, Type 2 diabetes, stroke and depression."[87] The most common type, obstructive sleep apnea, occurs when the throat muscles relax too much, and the inspiratory airway is sucked closed.

CPAP machines are designed to provide just enough air pressure to keep the upper airway passages from collapsing during sleep.

According to many of my clients, the mask can be uncomfortable and a challenge to keep clean. CPAP therapy is the reason so many families we know can't go camping with us anymore—inevitably, one of the partners needs electricity all night long, just to breathe! Thankfully, both oropharyngeal exercises and inspiratory muscle training rehabilitation interventions are applicable in rehabilitation programs for obstructive sleep apnea patients who do not accept CPAP therapy.[88]

Respiratory Muscle Training

In addition to CPAP machines, there are other effective treatment options. In a 2020 study, both oropharyngeal exercises (OE) and inspiratory muscle training (IMT) "leads [to] significant improvements in snoring severity and frequency, sleep quality, excessive daytime sleepiness, and the effect of sleepiness on daily life."[89] Training can also increase endurance in the inspiratory muscles. Segizbaey and colleagues (2014) note that "IMT elicits resistance to the development of inspiratory muscle fatigue during high-intensity exercise."[90] Further, core muscle function is also positively impacted by IMT. "Inspiratory muscle training can have a positive effect on core muscle function independent of specific core training."[91] Research has shown that respiratory muscle training increases respiratory muscle strength and endurance, and "these improvements result in reduced levels of breathlessness, and increase in predicted VO2 max and a perceived improvement in sports performance."[92]

Training load influences the response to inspiratory muscle training.[93] Functional inspiratory and core muscle training enhances running performance and economy.[94] Inspiratory muscle training improves the anti-reflux barrier in GERD patients.[95] Yoga is also effective. According to a systematic review and meta-analysis of the literature by Liu et al. (2014), limited "evidence suggested that yoga training has a positive effect on improving lung function and exercise capacity and could be used as an adjunct pulmonary rehabilitation program in COPD [chronic obstructive pulmonary disease] patients."[96] "The Pilates Method increases respiratory muscle strength,"[97] and yoga improved inspiratory muscle performance in veterans with COPD.[98] I recommend over-the-counter resisted-breathing devices to practice inspiratory muscle exercises for clients who snore.

Additionally, it should be noted that, in one study, a single manual therapy session with soft-tissue and joint mobilization "immediately improved pulmonary function, inspiratory muscle strength, and oxygen saturation and reduced dyspnea, fatigue, and heart and respiratory rates in patients with severe COPD."[99] The techniques used included myofascial release in the suboccipital area, sternocleidomastoid and trapezius muscles, intercostal and paravertebral muscles, and respiratory diaphragm. Joint mobilizations for gliding of the cervical, sternoclavicular, joint, scapulothoracic joint, thoracic vertebral articulations, and ribs were also performed. And in a different study, a single manual therapy session using soft tissue mobilization "appears to have the potential to produce immediate clinically meaningful improvements in lung function in patients with severe and very severe COPD."[100] This sounds like a normal manual therapy session to me! Again, we cannot separate the interconnected layers.

Hyperventilation

Studies reveal that "Both hyperventilation and upper chest breathing appear to be common patterns associated with pain."[101] This does not imply a causal relationship, just an association. Shelly Prosko summarizes that emotions affect breathing, and notes that "hyperventilation or breathing *too much* may actually be a stress response that occurs in situations where stress, fear and pain are uncontrollable."[102]

Emergency Core Muscles (Accessory Breathing Muscles)
Sympathetic Core Muscle Recruitment

The accessory breathing muscles of inspiration and expiration are over-recruited when the sustainable core muscles are not coordinated due to the demands of posture/gravity, IAP, or stress and pain. For this reason, I call the accessory breathing muscles the "emergency core muscles." Recall that the most common breathing disorder is *chest breathing*. In yoga, it is said that different types of breathing produce different mental states. Shallow breathing, or "Habitual chest breathing, not only reflects physical and mental problems, it creates them."[103] Physically, chest breathing over-recruits the accessory muscles of inspiration, including the pectoralis muscle.[104] Research by de Mayo et al. (2005) reveals that "Upper costal breathing type subjects showed a significantly higher suprahyoid EMG activity at rest than costo-diaphragmatic subjects in all body positions studied."[105] Diaphragm and external intercostal EMG activity suggests that there could be differences in motor unit recruitment strategies, depending on the breathing type.[106, 107] Clinical examination showed a characteristic pattern of standing, sitting, and walking, as well as lack of coordination and *irregular high costal respiration* in women with chronic pelvic pain.[108] Stress is correlated with an increase in muscle tension in the upper trapezius muscle,[109] and the intrinsic laryngeal muscle responds to stress.[110] Pain is associated with shallow breathing.

When our sustainable core muscles are unavailable for postural and breathing tasks, accessory breathing muscles are used to access our inspiratory reserve and our expiratory reserve volumes. It's important to access, exercise, or train our reserve muscular and breathing system for emergencies. However, it's not sustainable to always breathe with our reserve muscles, because "the accessory muscles are not designed to meet the needs of long-term independent ventilation and are more likely to fatigue and cause respiratory distress."[111] If we are constantly in a state of respiratory distress, our autonomic nervous system remains in a sympathetic nervous system state commonly called the "fight/flight/freeze" response.

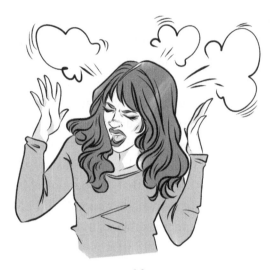

FIGURE 6.8 STRESS

The nervous system is divided into the central nervous system (CNS) and the peripheral nervous system (PNS). The CNS is composed of the spinal cord and the brain. The PNS is made of the nerves and other types of supporting cells that branch throughout the rest of the body and communicate back to the CNS.[112] The PNS is divided into the somatic nervous system and the autonomic nervous system (ANS), and the ANS is divided into the sympathetic nervous system, the parasympathetic nervous system, and the enteric nervous system. The somatic nervous system is divided into the sensory (afferent) and motor (efferent) inputs and outputs.[113]

In common terms, again, the sympathetic state is known as the "fight/flight/freeze" response, while the parasympathetic state is called the "rest and digest" response. Simply put, our body responds to threatening situations (real or perceived) by physiologically preparing for the next step of action. If we sense that a tiger is about to pounce on us, our heart rate increases, and blood flow is diverted away from digestion and repairing processes and is sent to the eyes (to see our threat better) and the muscles (in case we need to fight, "play dead," or run away from the threat).

The respiratory diaphragm muscle is a physical window into the state of our nervous system. When we are in the calm, parasympathetic state, we are peacefully using our RD to breathe. With every breath, the body is sending a constant signal to the brain via the RD that we are okay. The signals from the body to the brain can be termed "bottom-up" signals. The brain receives this information, processes it, and responds with a calm, passive exhalation, which perpetuates the state. However, when we demand more oxygen, or are startled, we recruit our accessory inhalation muscles or use a "chest breath." This change in recruitment of the muscles sends a different signal from the body to the brain: a signal that we might be in danger or that action is necessary. Our energy then shifts away from digestion and into muscle action. The three diaphragms are the coordinated switch center between the two states (see Figure 5.16).

Physical therapist and yoga therapist Matthew Taylor breaks this down in his simple educational videos about the three diaphragms.[114] He demonstrates how the three diaphragms impact stability and mobility of the body, and shows their relationship to the autonomic nervous system. Basically, when we are constantly or chronically in the fight or flight state, our bodies experience more pain, our mood elevators are depleted, our immune system is compromised, our balance is decreased, muscle tone increases, gastrointestinal function decreases, respiratory rate increases, heart rate increases, and quality of sleep and cognition are negatively affected.

Recall that pain is associated with faulty breathing.[115] Altered brain activity is detected during sustained muscle pain,[116] and it has also been shown that stress is a contributing factor to pain perception. "Current evidence suggests stress plays a contributing role in hyperalgesia and chronic pain."[117] Further, pain duration is associated with increased muscle sympathetic nerve activity.[118, 119] When we are constantly in a state of pain, discomfort, stress, fear, panic, or shallow breathing, we deprive our body of healing and proper metabolization of our food and oxygen.

Smith et al. determined that "Unlike obesity and physical activity, disorders of continence and respiration were strongly related to frequent back pain. This relationship may be explained by physiological limitations of co-ordination of postural, respiratory and continence functions of trunk muscles."[120] Perri concluded that "Based on this study, it can be suggested that evaluation and treatment of breathing pattern disorders must not be overlooked especially in the rehabilitation of chronic cervical pain."[121]

The body's physiological state affects the state of the breath. "Breathing mechanics are influenced directly by...Bio-mechanical factors such as rib head fixations or classical upper/lower crossed patterns of muscle imbalance."[122] Breathing mechanics are also affected by biochemical factors such as changes in pH balance (resulting from, e.g., allergy, infection, poor diet, hormonal influences, or kidney dysfunction), and psychosocial states such as chronic anxiety, anger, or depression.[123] In short, the respiratory diaphragm is the muscular switch station, or gate-keeper, between "rest and digest" and "fight or flight." We can measure this through vagal tone.

Vagal Tone

While the phrenic nerve innervates the respiratory diaphragm muscle, the vagus nerve is the relay switch with the RD between rest and digest and fight or flight. The vagus nerve, the tenth cranial nerve, is named for its wandering. It is really long! It emerges from the brain stem, travels down the neck, and sends branches to the larynx. It continues into the thorax, where it sends branches to the heart and lungs, and then pierces through the RD and innervates the intestinal organs. Vagal tone refers to the constant activity of the vagus nerve. Specifically, it refers to the continuous parasympathetic action that the vagus nerve exerts. Vagal tone is frequently used to assess heart function, and is also useful in assessing emotional regulation and other processes that alter, or are altered by, changes in parasympathetic activity.[124, 125] Research shows that yoga is correlated with both improvement in measures of psychological resilience[126] and improved vagal regulation.[127, 128, 129] Breit et al. (2018) emphasize that "vagal tone is correlated with capacity to regulate stress responses and can be influenced by breathing."[130]

Recall that different types of yogic breathing can affect the autonomic nervous system.[131] Shallow breathing is related to anxiety.[132] Luckily, yogic breathing techniques, where one lengthens the duration of the exhalation, are known to directly affect cardiac vagal tone.[133, 134, 135, 136, 137, 138] Specifically, "the practice of slow breathing exercise improves vagal activity."[139] We can use long, slow, soft complete exhalations to help us shift from a stressful nervous system state into the parasympathetic state. I find in the clinic that, when someone initially has difficulty properly engaging their TVA muscle, practicing and accomplishing a long, soft, slow, complete exhalation is a "way in" to help facilitate TVA control as well as calming the nervous system. Additionally, "deep breathing practice facilitates retention of newly learned motor skills."[140] Therefore, I recommend practicing various deep, slow, soft breathing exercises as homework for most clients seeking a sustainable core. The physical limb (*asana*) and breathing limbs (*pranayama*) of yoga are inseparable from any of the eight limbs.

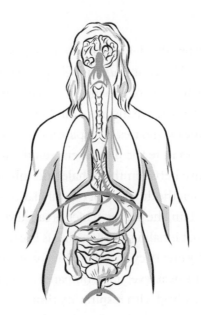

FIGURE 6.9 THE VAGUS NERVE

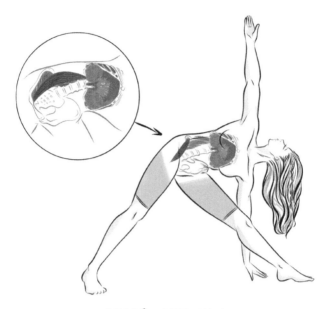

FIGURE 6.10 *TRIKONASANA*

Pranayama

In the yoga tradition, the definition of *pranayama* is "control of life (through breath)." The root *prana* is related to breath, or life, and *ayama* means to lengthen, or expand.[141] We can literally control our life force energy through expansion of our breath. We can dissect the breath cycle into the two phases of inspiration (*puraka*) and expiration (*recaka*). We also can note the pause between the inhale and exhale, as well as the pause between the exhale and inhale. Just as we can consciously lengthen the duration of our inhalation or exhalation, we can lengthen, or retain, the pauses, which is called *kumbhaka* in yoga. I often tell clients that inhaling and exhaling is Breathing 101. Knowing the four parts of the breath cycle (inhalation, pause, exhalation, pause) is Breathing 102 (the next level up). Compared to yoga breathing, deep breathing is not involved with respiratory timing changes, but rather focuses on breathing mechanics. "In contradistinction, the breathing technique of pranayama controls every phase of the breath, which is important for reducing anxiety and withdrawal symptoms before thoracic surgery."[142] The connection between breath, body, and spirit has long been understood in yoga. As Coulter notes, "Yogis…have discovered the value of regulating respiration consciously, of breathing evenly and diaphragmatically, of hyperventilating for specific purposes, and of suspending the breath at will."[143]

Consciously changing our breathing (and movement) patterns creates novelty, which our nervous system loves! Lengthening any of the four phases of the breath cycle can benefit our health. Specifically, lengthening the *exhalation* phase improves diaphragmatic function,[144] improves relaxation of the accessory inspiration muscles,[145] and increases parasympathetic activity.[146] Abdominal and yogic breathing have been shown to improve the symptoms of asthma[147] and COPD.[148, 149] In one investigation,[150] a 12-week yoga program improved a slew of breathing (and mental) metrics in young male medical student volunteers, not involved in any other athletic training program. The study yielded significant improvements in reaction times to light and sound, maximum expiratory pressure, maximum inspiratory pressure, 40 mmHg test, breath holding time after expiration, breath holding time after inspiration, and hand grip strength.[151]

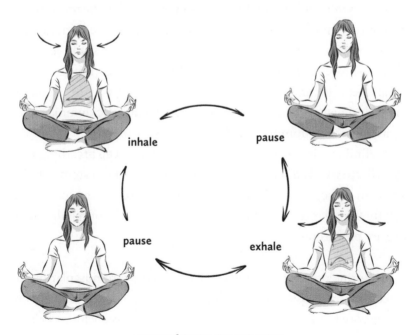

FIGURE 6.11 THE BREATH CYCLE

Bhramari pranayama—the "humming-bee breath"—and chanting OM are believed to be effective in improving pulmonary function in healthy individuals.[152] Studies have shown that breathing programs can help decrease low back pain[153, 154] and depression symptoms,[155] improve labor pain,[156] spinal curves,[157] and balance,[158] increase lung volume,[159] and improve memory,[160] cognition,[161] and quality of life.[162, 163] It is documented that breathing patterns affect sports performance,[164, 165] as well as posture, spinal stabilization, and motor control.[166, 167] Clinicians should include breathing exercises in the treatment of low back pain.[168] "The important link respiration has with health lies in its role as a doorway to the autonomic nervous system."[169]

Deep Slow Breathing

Specifically, regularly practiced *deep slow breathing* shows promise for positive changes in health and improvement in autonomic functions.[170] In a 2009 study[171] Jerath and Barnes found that "Deep slow breathing techniques lead to positive autonomic balance that affects brain, heart, and other organ systems innervated by the autonomic nervous system. It leads to drop in blood pressure and heart rate even without any meditative practice." These effects were even greater when combined with a meditative practice. In a later study, Jerath et al. (2015) proposed that "the ANS is modulated by breathing so that in sympathetic dominant states like stress and anxiety, slow-deep breathing techniques and meditation can shift sympathetic dominance to parasympathetic dominance."[172]

Preliminary investigation suggests that slow, deep breathing may contribute to a reduction in sympathetic nervous system activity and pain perception.[173] In addition, deep slow breathing may prove helpful to patients with fibromyalgia.[174] The results of regular practice are promising:

> Restoring proper breathing mechanics and neuromuscular motor control patterns during breathing may result in a decrease in pain, improved patient outcomes, and overall patient wellbeing associated with their primary musculoskeletal complaint. A comprehensive

evaluation of breathing patterns, as a part of an orthopedic examination, may guide a clinician in providing effective and appropriate treatments to decrease pain and improve function.[175]

Studies have measured the effects of deep, slow breathing on pain perception and autonomic activity. One such study suggests that "the way of breathing decisively influences autonomic and pain processing, thereby identifying DSB in concert with relaxation as the essential feature in the modulation of sympathetic arousal and pain perception."[176] Recall that meditation and deep slow breathing have been shown to help shift the ANS from sympathetic to parasympathetic dominance, and can be used as a primary treatment for anxiety.[177] This supports the idea that the "control switch" between the states of "fight or flight" and "rest and digest" could be the vagus nerve and the diaphragm.

Polyvagal Theory
Remember, the vagus nerve is long and has several branches. Some clinical psychologists and yoga therapists have popularized a theory that the branches serve an important role in emotional regulation, social connection, and fear response. For example, Porges' polyvagal theory (PVT)[178] proposes a mechanism called *neuroception* that triggers or inhibits defense strategies.[179] It holds that "Neuroception, as a process, determines whether specific features in the environment elicit specific physiological states that would support either fight–flight or social engagement behaviors."[180] "In PVT there are two vagal systems. The first is an evolved, mammalian, myelinated, ventral vagus [branch with...] pathways linked to [organs above the diaphragm.]" The second is "an older, reptilian un-myelinated, dorsal circuit that regulates the gut and sub diaphragmatic viscera."[181] "The identification of two vagal motor circuits, dorsal and ventral, provides an expanded understanding of stress response modulation."[182] Garner (2016) helps us apply Porges' work to this understanding. "Chiefly, if the CNS processes less motor input because the breath is at ease and not labored, then a yogic breath practice should improve stress response."[183]

"It is proposed that...yoga-based interventions support the return towards optimal balance [by improving] function...in regions of the brain that regulate response to threat," which helps reduce allostatic load.[184] These findings underscore the fact that "The diaphragm is the key connecting point of the two vagal pathways."[185]

When clients arrive in the studio in "fight or flight" mode, I find they are often simply unable to learn new movement tasks. My first aid for these clients is to regain conscious control of their diaphragms. Studies, such as the one by Bordoni et al. (2013), support this reasoning: the functions of the diaphragm do not stop locally in its anatomy but affect the whole body system.[186] We start with the breath. "Breathing practices can be an accessible, easy, safe and effective treatment strategy to modulate pain that can give the person in pain a sense of self-efficacy and empowerment in their pain care."[187] This clinical practice has been borne out by the research. "The potential for improving the patient's state, by optimizing their breathing pattern in all their activities, is an important development in physiotherapy. It is a developing area of knowledge which is pertinent to physiotherapy practice as it develops in a bio-psychosocial model."[188]

Now that we understand all the benefits of efficient and resilient breathing patterns, let's learn about some specific breathing exercises (you can find instructions for most of the discussed exercises in Part III).

Abdomino-Diaphragmatic Breath (Calming Breath)

In all of my trained disciplines, the abdomino-diaphragmatic breath is considered the gold standard for relaxation (see Figure 6.5). Expanding the RD into a soft or nonrestricted abdomen allows the muscle to reach its full range of motion potential. I use it as a window into the state of the nervous system, and a way out of the sympathetic nervous system's "fight or flight" response into the parasympathetic nervous system's "rest and digest" response.[189] My first practical experience with this breathing intervention came instinctively.

When I was a young student athletic trainer, I was driving an athlete to an off-campus doctor's appointment in the college van. She was sitting in the passenger seat and suddenly started to panic. She was visibly having difficulty breathing. I heard the pitch of her breath increase and could tell that her airways were restricted. She was having an asthma attack! I pulled over and helped her get her inhaler. I could see that she was using her chest, shoulder, and neck muscles to gasp for more air. I intuitively found myself instructing her to inhale the medicine deeply into the lower lobes of her lungs "as if you could breathe into your belly."

This was before I had any yoga training, and before I knew what "belly breathing" was. It was visibly obvious to me that she was in a state of panic and that she was hyperventilating and overtaxing her upper chest muscles. I had never seen anyone breathe like that before. Instinctively, I knew it wasn't good! She was able to gain control quickly before I felt it necessary to call for additional help on the university police walkie talkie—this was before cell phones.

Later, I saw this chest/panic breath when a close friend was having a panic attack. I didn't know what a panic attack was then; to me, it looked like the college athlete's asthma attack. My friend (who prefers the pronouns they/them) had the same chest breathing and visibly taxed neck and shoulder muscles as the athlete had exhibited. This time I had some experience. Without thinking, I instructed them in the same way I had instructed the athlete: to breathe deeply and calmly into their lower body. This time, I also told them that they were safe and that they had the power to control their own breathing. I used rhythm and counting as a focal redirect, and reminded them that they were in control of their body, and they had the power to slow...their...breath...down. It worked!

In both cases, encouraging the person to focus inward, empowering them to regain self-control, and attempting to expand their respiratory diaphragm muscle helped them overcome their difficulties breathing.

The abdomino-diaphragmatic breath is performed with abdominal muscles relaxed. In this condition the central tendon of the RD is mobile, and "the diaphragm's origin (the base of the ribcage) is stable."[190] In other words, the central tendon is the moving anchor, and the rib cage appears still. When the abdominal muscles are relaxed, the intestines, pelvic organs, and PFM get displaced downward, and the abdominal muscles stretch outward. The visible motion occurs in the abdomen (while the chest, spine, and ribs are still). In sitting and standing positions, the respiratory diaphragm muscle is assisted by gravity during inhalation. When the body is parallel to the ground (face up or face down), the RD is not resisted by gravity; kinesiologists term this a "gravity neutral" position. When we are inverted, like in a handstand or downward-facing dog pose, the RD is gravity resisted (or it has to work harder against the force of gravity). In any position relative to gravity, the fibers of the RD shorten on the inhalation (concentric contraction) and the central tendon is the moving part. This calming breath, with the TVA relaxed, is often called a "belly breath" because the belly is where the visible motion occurs. I prescribe this breath for promoting relaxation. Please see the specific instructions for belly breathing in Part III of this book.

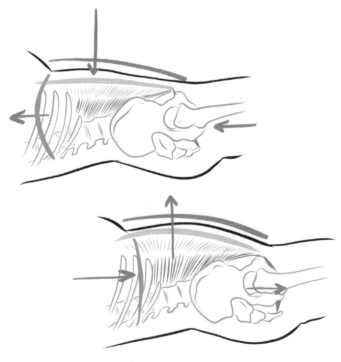

FIGURE 6.12 SUPINE BELLY BREATH

While belly breathing is a great relaxation strategy, fully relaxing the transverse abdominis muscle does not provide efficient dynamic core spinal stability for movement tasks. In other words, belly breathing is not the technique I recommend for breathing during sports or high-load activities. Instead, I recommend providing a little tension in the glottis or TVA to dynamically stabilize the spine. When we do this, we effectively flip the origin and insertion of the respiratory diaphragm muscle and can continue to breathe diaphragmatically, while engaging our sustainable core muscles. This is called a thoraco-diaphragmatic breath.

Thoraco-Diaphragmatic Breath (Centering Breath)

Full expansion of the diaphragmatic muscle is still possible with contraction of the deep abdominal muscles. When the TVA is engaged, the abdominal cavity becomes more rigid and stable. This rigidity packages the intestines together and the diaphragm muscle cannot descend into the abdominal cavity. Instead, it bumps into the rigidly held abdominal organs, and the abdominal organs can't be compressed, so they act as a cantilever and the base of the rib cage expands like an umbrella.[191] "If the central tendon is stabilized, and the ribs are free to move, a diaphragmatic contraction will cause an expansion of the ribcage."[192] *The origin and insertion of the respiratory diaphragm muscle are functionally flipped.* Even though there is a little belly bulging or expansion, the lateral thoracic breath primarily utilizes the diaphragm muscle and produces anterior, posterior, *and* lateral costal expansion. The central tendon becomes the stable attachment, and the base of the rib cage becomes the visible moving part. In thoraco-diaphragmatic breath (also known as lateral thoracic breath or lateral costal breath), the TVA or glottis are engaged, and the diaphragm expands fully.

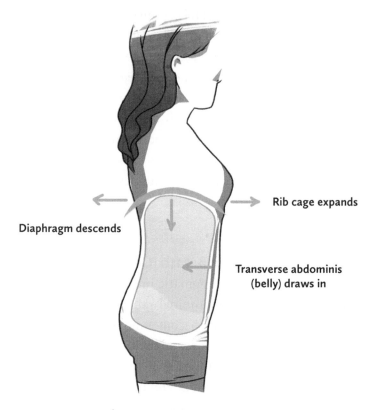

Rib cage expands

Diaphragm descends

Transverse abdominis
(belly) draws in

FIGURE 6.13 THORACO-DIAPHRAGMATIC BREATH

This breath pattern has many other names. I learned it first in Pilates simply as a "Pilates breath." "In the Pilates method, the respiratory style accentuates costal breathing, where the ribs ascend and descend during the respiratory flow, extending laterally and to the posterior."[193] In the Z-Health method, it is called a band breath.[194] In the Medical Therapeutic Yoga model, it is called a TATD (transverse abdominis assisted thoraco-diaphragmatic) breath,[195] and physical therapist Julie Wiebe calls it an umbrella breath.[196] I find that clients can readily visualize an umbrella, mushroom, or jellyfish fairly well when they recognize the three-dimensional aspect of the respiratory diaphragm muscle. Combining these visualizations with the tactile input of an elastic exercise band or their hands can also be helpful learning tools.

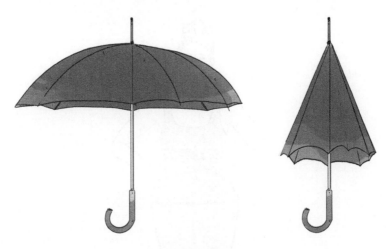

FIGURE 6.14 UMBRELLA

When taxed with limb movement, the thoraco-diaphragmatic breath is the ideal combination of core stability and efficient oxygen exchange. This is a breath I encourage people to explore anytime we are not consciously relaxing the abdominal muscles. This is the breath that I teach the most, and once accomplished, it *can* change lives. Yogis call this breath centering and I witness energetic shifts when people find the balance between engaging their sustainable core muscles while fully utilizing their RD's full potential range of movement. In fitness circles it is called a "band breath" because we can place an elastic exercise band around the thorax for tactile input. (Please see the specific instructions for thoraco-diaphragmatic breathing in Chapter 10, Breathing Exercises.)

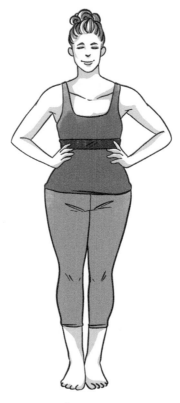

FIGURE 6.15 BAND BREATH

Both the thoraco-diaphragmatic and abdomino-diaphragmatic breaths are "diaphragmatic breaths." One engages the TVA. One does not. In the abdomino-diaphragmatic breath, the belly expands. The thoraco-diaphragmatic breath causes the rib cage to expand laterally. This is not to be confused with a chest breath, where elevation of the rib cage occurs. And recall that a chest breath can trigger us, via the vagus nerve, to put us in an excited state. "Hyperventilation is often characterized by a shift from a diaphragmatic to a thoracic breathing pattern, which imposes biomechanical stress on the neck/shoulder region due to the ancillary recruitment of sternocleidomastoid, scalene, and trapezius muscles in support of thoracic breathing."[197] We don't want to practice or perpetuate that kind of breathing in a panic state. However, we do want to be prepared for an emergency.

Three-Part Breath (*Dirga Pranayama*—Full, Yogic Breath)

Every muscle needs full length and strength to perform daily tasks. Just like we train our muscles to get stronger for an athletic event, we can train the muscles that help us breathe. We can *strengthen* the accessory breathing muscles with resistance (e.g., inspiratory muscle training) and resisted exhaling (blowing up a balloon or blowing through a straw). How do we stretch the breathing muscles? With *pranayama* exercises focused on increasing the inspiratory reserve volume in the chest and thorax.

Dirga pranayama, a three-part breath, combines the abdomino-diaphragmatic breath, the thoraco-diaphragmatic breath, and a little chest breath in a safe environment. I prescribe this breath to stretch the accessory inhalation muscles. We can lengthen or stretch the emergency breathing muscles (in this case the inspiratory reserve muscles) with intention. I often teach this breath to clients who have rigid or tight upper thoracic muscles or stiff or hypomobile thoracic and costal joints, chronic chest breathers, and people who could benefit from increased lung capacity. I recommend practicing it in a quiet, comfortable environment, or when they are in the parasympathetic (rest and digest) state, to encourage a "bottom up" signal of safety to the brain.

One study used three-part breath before and after trauma-releasing exercises as an effective intervention in a program designed to help social workers and other health professionals learn effective self-directed techniques to address the incidence of secondary trauma and post-traumatic stress disorder.[198] Another study showed that three-part breath improved upper extremity function and scapular posturing in persons with hyperkyphosis.[199]

A more recent study showed that a yogic breath was superior to standard breathing exercises in preparing lung cancer patients for surgery.[200] In this case, the yogic breath used was a combination of a belly breath and a thoracic breath to purposefully employ the accessory breathing muscles. The researchers' instructions to the participants included "Respiration should be accompanied by a sense of calmness. In addition, patients were asked to focus on extending expiration to counteract air trapping in the lungs and to slow expiratory flow."[201] In other words, they lengthened the duration of the exhalation and instructed the participants to go slowly. I believe that the instructions to go slowly were so as not to induce an excited state in the participants.

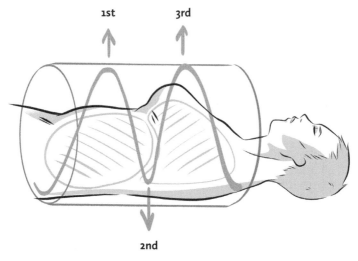

FIGURE 6.16 *DIRGA PRANAYAMA*

This breath is sometimes referred to as a "complete breath" because we completely "fill" our inspiratory reserve capacity. Alternately, it is called a "wave breath" due to the wave of motion created by the visible change in volume from the bottom up during the inhalation. *Dirga* means three, but this breath can be divided into two parts (as in the lung cancer study) or, theoretically, into thousands of parts. Another way to explore the three-part breath is to think about expanding and relaxing the three diaphragms in sequence during the inhalation:

1. Inhale into the relaxed pelvis and PFM (reverse Kegel)
2. Continue the inhalation into the relaxed belly and thorax (abdomino-diaphragmatic plus thoraco-diaphragmatic breath)
3. Continue inhaling into the relaxed throat and glottis muscles.

Once you master the relaxation of the three diaphragms on the inhalation, I recommend exploring controlling the glottis on the inhale and exhale. Controlled glottal breathing is called *ujjayi pranayama*[202] or "victorious breath."

Ujjayi Breath (Controlled Glottal Breathing)

Recall that glottal control influences balance,[203] and the glottis forms the pressure valve at the top of the core cylinder (see Figure 5.15).[204] During respiration, a slight contraction of the laryngeal muscles and partial closure of the glottis produces an "ocean" or "rushing" sound, due to the partial closure of the throat space. In yoga this is an *ujjayi*, or "victorious," breath sound. Also called "hissing breath" or "psychic breath," this *pranayama* technique has many health benefits.

During an *exhalation*, the laryngeal muscles concentrically contract to produce the sound. When we constrict or maintain this closure during an *inhalation*, the muscles are eccentrically contracting. *Ujjayi* breathing increases the pressure of air on the lungs and strengthens the glottal opening. Practicing *Ujjayi* breath is essentially the same thing as eccentrically strengthening the muscles in the vocal folds. Yoga "incorporates various exercises of breathing, oropharyngeal structures and facial expressions the physiology and effect of which are comparable to international physiotherapy recommendations in treatment of obstructive sleep apnea," for example "to preserve upper airway patency by maintaining airway dilator muscle tone."[205] In other words, eccentrically strengthening the glottal opening prevents it from collapsing under increased pressure on an inhalation. This is why *ujjayi* breath can improve the symptoms of sleep apnea; stronger muscles stay open and are more resilient to the changing demands of inhalation during a relaxed state. In addition to improving sleep apnea,[206, 207, 208] *ujjayi* breath decreases snoring, helps asthma, affects thyroid and parathyroid gland function, and has even been shown to offset the effects of bone loss and osteoporosis in astronauts.[209] "An increase of 19% in oxygen consumption has been observed during the practice of one type of pranayama called the *ujjayi pranayama.*"[210] Another study demonstrated that *ujjayi pranayama* training combined with medical treatment and diaphragmatic breathing exercise improves lung vital capacity measures in patients with mild bronchial asthma.[211] "*Ujjayi* breathing is safe and beneficial for most bipolar patients because it is calming as opposed to stimulating... *Ujjayi* quiets the mind, reduces obsessive worry, and induces a state of physical and mental calmness conducive to sleep."[212]

According to yoga teacher Aadil Palkhivala, the sound of *ujjayi pranayama* serves two purposes:

> One, it stimulates the *nadis*, or energy channels, in the sinuses and at the back of the throat. This, in turn, promotes mental clarity and focus. It also provides a sound to latch onto, so that the mind can become more still. When the sound oscillates, the mind too is oscillating, and the student can hear this.[213]

As a teacher, the sound offers a window into the student's mind.

Three Diaphragms and Energy

Thus far, we have discussed the three diaphragm muscles (PFM, RD, and glottis) as part of the sustainable core (see Figure 5.16). We have examined their inseparability from each other insofar as the PFM and RD move parallel to each other like a piston. We have determined that breathing is much more effective during contraction of the PFM.[214] We have also investigated the fact that the three diaphragm muscles respond to resilience training, just like any other muscle group in the body. In Part III of this book I offer instructions for gentle *pranayama* practices that stimulate these muscles and are accessible to most bodies (see the box "Tetraplegia").

Tetraplegia

For those bodies with tetraplegia (a complete severance injury to the spinal cord at the C5–C6 level or lower), the connection, or nerve innervation, to the pelvic floor and abdominal muscles is cut through entirely. Typically, this population will be using an abdominal binder which "results in significant improvements in respiratory function for individuals with tetraplegic SCI [spinal cord injury]."[215] Using an abdominal binder is thought to restore abdominal pressure and consequently improve breathing capacity and reduce postural hypotension in patients who do not have functioning abdominal muscles. Tetraplegia can manifest with many different muscle scenario presentations, but if the injury is below the C5–C6 level, the glottis, trapezius, and diaphragm muscles should still be accessible, albeit very weak. *Pranayama* exercises will continue to facilitate neuromuscular connection and strengthen these muscles, and glottal strategies along with an abdominal binder are recommended for upper body core control.

Exploring the Breathing Core

Once we establish central alignment and voluntary coordination of the sustainable core muscles, the foundation is set for accomplishing the thoraco-diaphragmatic breath, or umbrella breath. It is a main goal of mine to help people breathe with more diaphragm muscle range of motion while maintaining dynamic control of their sustainable core muscles during activity. This is what is happening during the umbrella breath. I ask yoga practitioners and endurance athletes if they are consciously able to shift to a combination of thoraco-diaphragmatic and controlled glottal breathing when times get tough. If not, that becomes a goal.

Now that you understand that the aim of the individual practices is to gain control over the coordination of the core with the breath, I recommend exploring the different breathing exercises in this chapter. Here is an example of instructions I might give to someone who has demonstrated good control of the RD with and without the TVA engaged:

- *Exhale* and lightly engage your pelvic floor muscles and transverse abdominis muscle, downwardly rotate your shoulder blades (engage your wings), and "extend your crown." (By "lightly" I mean "less than moderately," or about 10%–30% of a maximal contraction.)
- Maintain the lifting action of the skull and the scapular position while you continue to breathe in and out.
- Continue to lightly contract the PFM and TVA muscles (with the exhale) and release the muscle tension (with the inhale) in rhythm with your breath, ideally while your wings maintain your scapular position in space.
- Explore the ranges of motion of the PFM and TVA with the breath, without changing your bony core position, for 6–10 breath cycles.
- Once this is accomplished, try combining the reverse Kegel breath with the TVA contraction and relaxation, *and* work on expanding the range of motion of the posterior thorax with the thoraco-diaphragmatic breathing exercise. You will find instructions for all three of these individual exercises in Chapters 10 and 11.

The gentle breathing practices I have introduced so far (breath awareness, lengthening the exhalation, abdomino-diaphragmatic breath, thoraco-diaphragmatic breath, three-part breath, and controlled glottal breath/*ujjayi pranayama*) are also gateways to the energetic core. The three diaphragms are one set of keys to unlock this connection. (I provide specific instructions for exploring and practicing these breaths in Chapter 10.) They are my first choices for helping clients rehabilitate their bodies, and for clients with *most* musculoskeletal dysfunctions. In my experience, if one does not have automatic control of their sustainable core muscles in their daily movements, less efficient muscles take over, substitute, and work "harder" than they have to. This is a sufficient strategy in an emergency, but relying on the limbs or accessory breathing muscles for repetitive or high-load activities is not sustainable in daily life. Ideally, we want the muscles of the arms and legs, and the reserve lung volumes (IRV and ERV), to be ready for more demanding tasks. In the studio, I can't help clients learn new movement patterns until they are aware of their habitual and inefficient movement patterns.

The first step in any breathing practice is cultivating self-aware-ness. In her 2022 book *Yoga for Times of Change*, Nina Zolotow sug-gests breath *awareness* as a primary intervention for stress relief.[216] Accordingly, my job as a movement therapist is not so different from that of a psychotherapist. Psychotherapists offer mental counseling to help clients learn and practice healthier thought patterns and social behaviors. Physical therapists offer practices to help clients learn more efficient (and often less painful) movement patterns. In order to change our habits, we have to become aware of our ineffi-ciencies. Just as in yoga philosophy, removing obstacles, or *kleshas*, to liberation, peace, and freedom is part of the practice.[217]

7

THE MINDFUL CORE

The word *klesha* in Sanskrit means "painful affliction" or "to poison." The term is used to denote specific negative mental patterns that obscure our true nature and are considered to be the cause of suffering in yogic and Buddhist philosophy.[1] According to Patanjali's *Yoga Sutra*, the five *kleshas* are *avidya* (ignorance), *asmita* (egoism or I-am-ness), *raga* (attachment), *dvesha* (repulsion and aversion), and *abhinivesha* (fear of death and the will to live).[2] Perhaps the easiest of these to understand initially is *avidya*; it reminds me of the saying "Ignorance is bliss." If we don't know what is causing us harm, we might continue to ignore our body's early warning signs of dis-ease until sickness overcomes us. While I practice non-dogmatic philosophy, I do believe that getting to the root of a patient's suffering is part of the job description in musculoskeletal rehabilitation.

Yogic philosophy can be helpful in cultivating compassion for yourself and helping clients ease their suffering. Gaining a sense of the client's self-awareness can be extremely helpful in guiding them through unfamiliar or scary movements. Emotions affect breathing and pain.[3] Breathing patterns change with pain. While Western science has yet to "prove" why yoga "works," we are solidifying the understanding that it is multifactorial, and understanding the philosophy itself is a step in the healing process.

Why Does Yoga Work?

Remember, yoga is correlated both with improvement in measures of psychological resilience[4] and improved vagal regulation.[5, 6, 7] Briet et al. (2018) observe that "vagal tone is correlated with capacity to regulate stress responses and can be influenced by breathing."[8] But how?

In a 2022 study, researchers asked, "Do physical therapy and yoga improve pain and disability through psychological mechanisms?"[9] In the limited study, they found that "Improvements in perceived stress mediated improvements in disability after PT treatment compared to education. Other psychological outcomes did not mediate the effect of yoga or PT on pain or disability outcomes compared to education."[10] So, why does yoga work? Recall that the attempt to squeeze yoga philosophy into the allopathic medical paradigm is reductionist and dualistic.

Ernst (2017) states that "In principle, the reductionist approach assumes that if scientists investigate every part of the human body and its possible interactions with other parts and when they put it all together, they will understand human physiology."[11] But we know that physiology is interactive, and that humans are more complex than that.

The BPSS model is integrative, not reductionist. We can influence the brain with the body (termed "bottom-up" signals) and we can influence the body with the brain ("top-down" signals). The pathways from the brain to the gut and the intestines to the brain are a two-way street. These pathways include the neuro-anatomical, immunological, neuroendocrine hypothalamic–pituitary axis, neurotransmitters, neuropeptides, and microbial-derived products. "Mind-body therapies, including yoga therapy, are proposed to benefit health and well-being through integration of top-down and bottom-up processes facilitating bidirectional communication between the brain and body."[12] Examples of "top-down" regulation in a movement practice are regulation of attention and setting of intention. Sullivan et al. (2018) relate that these are "shown to decrease psychological stress as well as hypothalamic-pituitary axis (HPA) and sympathetic nervous system (SNS) activity, and in turn modulate immune function and inflammation."[13] Furthermore, it should be acknowledged that bottom-up regulation is promoted by breathing and movement practices, and are "shown to influence the musculoskeletal, cardiovascular and nervous system function and also affect HPA and SNS activity with concomitant changes in immune function and emotional well-being."[14]

We can use movement to influence any aspect of one's existence (because movement can change emotions, mind, and breath), and we can use psychology to influence any aspect of existence![15] In other words, we don't have to rely on the use of the body to change the body or the mind to change the mind; we can use any aspect of existence to change any aspect of existence. "The reductionist approach does not appreciate the tight interconnection of different parts of the body to function in real time."[16] Our language matters, and the evolving field of yoga therapy is attempting to acknowledge this while honoring the roots of yoga.

The International Association of Yoga Therapists defines yoga therapy as "the process of empowering individuals to progress toward improved health and well-being through the application of the teachings and practices of yoga."[17] In yoga therapy, the emphasis is not on symptom suppression, but rather on the client's journey of discovering the source of their suffering (*duhkha*), facilitating ease, and cultivating well-being (*salutogenesis*).

> *Salutogenesis* is an emphasis on client care that identifies and addresses the causes of health/well-being with interventions focused on health promotion and optimizing well-being... This shift in perspective is a key difference from the pathology-focused care in our culture... Yoga therapy focuses on health promotion and well-being, not pathology.[18]

Yoga therapy is *not* the application of yogic tools for symptom management of a diagnosis made by another health care provider. That is termed *yogaopathy*, where "the suffix 'pathy' implies a focus on disease and pathogenesis" with a segmented approach as opposed to an integrated one.[19] Yoga therapy is a process, not an outcome, and that is difficult to reproduce in the laboratory. Nonetheless, this perspective *is* what my clients have asked me to share, and put into words. The journey is individual and unique.

Two of the many possible reasons the process of yoga therapy "works" are through promoting resilience and self-regulation. *Self-regulation* is:

> a conscious ability to maintain stability of the system by managing or altering responses to threat or adversity, [which] may reduce symptoms of diverse conditions such as irritable bowel syndrome, neurodegenerative conditions, chronic pain, depression and PTSD through the mitigation of allostatic load with an accompanying shift in autonomic state.[20]

Resilience "includes the ability of an individual to 'bounce back' and adapt in response to adversity and/or stressful circumstances in a timely way such that psychophysiological resources are conserved."[21] *High* resilience "is correlated with quicker cardiovascular recovery following subjective emotional experiences…, less perceived stress, greater recovery from illness or trauma and better management of dementia and chronic pain," while "*Compromised* resilience is linked to *dysregulation* of the autonomic nervous system through measures of vagal regulation" (emphasis added).[22]

Recall from Sullivan et al. (2018) that yoga therapy informed by philosophical and ethical perspectives provides "a lens through which to understand how yogic practices support the individual's transformation in the experience of illness, pain, or disability."[23] The authors propose "that this transformation occurs through facilitating a reharmonization of body, mind, and environment toward the experience of eudaimonic well-being."[24] Interestingly, Sullivan et al. say that:

> The concept of *eudaimonia*, often defined as a life well-lived or well-intentioned, can further elucidate the benefits of cultivating

a life of meaning and purpose for both subjective well-being and physiological health. Thus far, the problem explored has been phenomenological, working with the LB/LE [lived body or lived experience] of pain or disability. Reconciliation can be explored through the concept of eudaimonic well-being or a well-lived life of fulfilled meaning and purpose. **Yoga therapy then becomes the path and practice toward the ultimate aim of a life of meaning and purpose in the realization of well-being.** (Emphasis added)[25]

With this in mind, we can also understand some of the neurophysiological explanations about how yoga supports various populations and conditions. Ray, Pathak, and Tomer (2011) note, "Although yogic practices are low intensity exercises within lactate threshold, physical performance improvement is possible owing to both better economy of breathing by [breathing maneuvers] and also by improvement in cardiovascular reserve. Other factors such as psycho-physiological and better relaxation may contribute."[26] In addition, the mechanisms involved include regulation of the nervous and endocrine systems, mood, and emotions.[27] The mechanisms which link these various aspects of practice include regulation of allostatic load[28] and polyvagal theory.[29]

While we have already mentioned polyvagal theory in its neurophysiological context:

> PVT can be conceptualized as a neurophysiological counterpart to the yogic concept of the *gunas*, or qualities of nature. Similar to the neural platforms described in PVT, the *gunas* provide the foundation from which behavioral, emotional and physical attributes emerge... these two different yet analogous frameworks—one based in neurophysiology and the other in an ancient wisdom tradition—highlight yoga therapy's promotion of physical, mental and social wellbeing for self-regulation and resilience.[30]

We will briefly discuss the *gunas* shortly.

Allostatic load refers to the cumulative burden of chronic stress and life events.[31] Recall that "vagal tone is correlated with capacity to regulate stress responses and can be influenced by breathing."[32] For this reason, "Yoga practice is intrinsically tailored to promote vagal tone and reduce allostatic load in several ways. First, slow and rhythmic breathing (especially when performed with increased airway resistance) promotes activation of the parasympathetic nervous system and increases HRV [heart rate variability]."[33]

Heart Rate Variability and Vagal Tone

Heart rate variability (HRV) is the term used to describe a state where the amount of time between heartbeats fluctuates slightly.[34] HRV is suggested to be a reliable assessment of autonomic function, an index of cardiovascular adaptability, and indicative of autonomic or sympatho-vagal balance.[35, 36, 37, 38] In other words, *HRV is an indicator of vagal tone*. There are several methods available to measure cardiac autonomic nervous system capacity, and heart rate variability has been established as one of these measures with the advantage of being a noninvasive tool. "Classical spectral analysis of HRV signals distinguishes sympathetic from the parasympathetic activity."[39] Basically, having a high variation in heart rate reflects the heart's resilience, and high variability is healthier. "Low HRV is a risk factor for pathophysiology and psychopathology,"[40] and is associated with low vagal tone.[41, 42] Heart rate variability fluctuations can "indicate current or future health problems, including heart conditions and mental health issues like anxiety and depression."[43] They are "frequently introduced as mirroring imbalances within the autonomous nerve system."[44] There have been several experimental investigations "based on the paradigm that increased sympathetic tone is associated with decreased parasympathetic tone and *vice versa*."[45] Increasing vagal tone activates the parasympathetic nervous system, and having higher vagal tone means that the body can relax faster after stressful events. HRV is an accessible way to measure our physical and psychological resilience.

Many studies[46] have reported the HRV of *pranayama* practices before and after the practice, but only very few studies have reported the HRV *during* the *pranayama* practices such as alternate nostril breathing[47] and *kapalabhati*.[48, 49] "Heart rate variability changes during and after the practice of *bhramari pranayama*."[50]

Yoga practice also promotes vagal tone and reduced allostatic load by enhancing the depth of the breath, "thus boosting the effects of the breathing practices themselves."[51] Additionally, "postures that emphasize abdominal tone through interior muscle activation additionally promote peripheral vagal stimulation and afference."[52] Finally, "attempting to maintain a slow and steady breathing rhythm during physical, mental, and emotional challenges elicited by the yoga practice itself represents an opportunity to practice nonreactive awareness and cultivate a state of equanimity in the face of stress."[53]

What effects do breathing techniques have? "Breathing techniques are known to directly affect cardiac vagal tone and the initiation of the vagal brake to move the system towards the [ventral vagal complex] platform and provides another bottom-up regulatory practice of yoga."[54] The bottom line is that *yoga allows us to rehearse and practice healthier responses to stress and adverse situations, both physically and mentally.* When we physically challenge ourselves by twisting and bending near our end-ranges or physical limits, we trigger a neurological stress response state. But, when we are consciously aware that we are near the edge of control, we can back off the edge, tune inwardly toward our breath and bodily sensations, and practice how to down-train the stress response in a safe environment. HRV and biofeedback training "may be a promising intervention to improve pain catastrophizing and the psychological responses of injured athletes throughout the rehabilitation process."[55]

HRV gives us a window into how the brain, heart, and gut communicate. "A low vagal tone, as assessed by heart rate variability, a marker of the sympatho-vagal balance, is observed in functional digestive disorders and inflammatory bowel diseases."[56] The vagus nerve may play a role in the inflammation process. "This vagal function is mediated through several pathways. The first one is the anti-inflammatory hypothalamic–pituitary–adrenal axis which is stimulated by vagal afferent fibres and leads to the release of cortisol by the adrenal glands and efferent (activation of the CAP) fibres."[57]

Gut–Brain Axis

"The vagus nerve constantly sends updated sensory information about the state of the body's organs 'upstream' to your brain via afferent nerves. In fact, 80 to 90 percent of the nerve fibers in the vagus nerve are dedicated to communicating the state of your viscera up to your brain."[58] "The gut-brain axis refers to the two-way connection and communication between the gut and the brain. What is happening in the gut can directly influence our brain function and behaviour."[59] And vice versa!

Because of its position as a key element of the autonomic nervous system in gut–brain interactions, the vagus nerve "seems to be a good therapeutic target in inflammatory conditions of the digestive tract (e.g. IBD) and also other inflammatory conditions such as [rheumatoid arthritis], and others."[60] Evidence indicates that gut microbiota can also influence the immune and nervous systems and vice versa.[61, 62, 63, 64] The vagus nerve is a main communicator in the gut–brain axis, and stress has a huge influence.[65, 66]

Interoception

How do you feel? This "gut" sense of how we are doing is termed *interoception*, or the sense of the physical condition of the body, especially sensations arising from the viscera.[67] "Interoception is a process consisting of integrating the information coming from the inside of the body in the central nervous system and the appreciation that complex emotional processes are fundamentally affected by the processing and regulation of somatic states."[68] In short, "Interoception is the perception of sensations from inside the body and includes the perception of physical sensations related to internal organ function such as heartbeat, respiration, satiety, as well as the autonomic nervous system activity related to emotions."[69]

Pain is a form of interoception:

Negative emotions are associated with increased activation in the amygdala, anterior cingulate cortex, and anterior insula – these brain structures not only mediate the processing of emotions, but are also important nodes of the pain neuromatrix that tune attention toward pain, intensify pain unpleasantness, and amplify interoception.[70]

Research indicates that "Disrupted interoception is a prominent feature of the diagnostic classification of several psychiatric disorders."[71] "Recent functional anatomical work has detailed an afferent neural system in primates and in humans that represents all aspects of the physiological condition of the physical body. This system constitutes a representation of 'the material me', and might provide a foundation for subjective feelings, emotion and self-awareness."[72] Finally, "Altered breathing may be useful as a physiological marker of anxiety as well as a treatment target using interoceptive interventions."[73]

In some studies, paced slow breathing is associated with pain reduction, "but evidence elucidating the underlying physiological mechanisms of this effect is lacking."[74] However, there is evidence that "Volitional pacing of the breath engages fronto-temporal-insular cortices, whereas attention to automatic breathing modulates the cingulate cortex [in the brain]."[75] Notably, "the core of the definition of interoception is on the subjective experience above all else; thus we can say the brain is the true source, i.e., the real origin of interoception."[76] In short, pain is interpreted in the brain, and we can learn how to respond to sensations in new ways. I tell clients that one of our goals is to have a more loving, two-way conversation between their body and mind. Their symptoms are their body's way of speaking up—we have to listen to our bodies to understand what they need before we can make those changes. Often, when we make changes, the symptoms change, too.

"The core task of a brain working in service to the body is allostasis: regulating the body's internal systems by anticipating needs and preparing to satisfy them before they arise. Interoception—your brain's representation of sensations from your own body—is the sensory consequence of this activity."[77] Mindfulness is a practice that helps us cultivate interoception.[78]

Mindfulness

Yoga includes mindfulness, and mindfulness-based stress reduction (MBSR) techniques in psychology include yoga. Both practices are known to help reduce pain and incorporate mindfulness techniques.[79] "Mindful awareness has been defined as 'the awareness that emerges through paying attention on purpose, in the present moment, and nonjudgmentally to the unfolding experience, moment by moment.'"[80] Linda Carlson reminds us that cultivation of mindfulness "is both a practice and a way of being in the world."[81] "For millenniums, mindfulness was believed to diminish pain by reducing the influence of self-appraisals of noxious sensations."[82] "Through mindful breathing, body scan, and movement, patients build body awareness and learn to sense and interpret bodily sensations in new, non-threatening ways."[83] The most recent evidence, as noted by Reigner et al. in 2022, proposes that mindfulness meditation-induced pain relief might be associated with "a novel self-referential nociceptive gating mechanism to reduce pain."[84] Pain is interpreted in the brain and mindfulness training can help us modulate it.

"Mindfulness training actively engages patients in pain self-management within a biopsychosocial framework"[85] which fits within the recommendations for chronic pain management by the American Interagency Pain Research Coordinating Committee (IPRCC).[86] The IPRCC states, "Self-management programs can improve quality of life and are an important component of acute and chronic pain prevention and management."[87]

Joe Tatta and colleagues (2022) urge that "The Time Is Now" to incorporate mindfulness-based therapies in physical therapist practice.[88] They note that mindfulness and acceptance based interventions are associated with improved health outcomes such as "physical function, injury prevention, pain management, immune function, and noncommunicable diseases."[89] Additionally, studies have shown that "MBSR is a promising adjunctive therapy for IC/BPS [interstitial cystitis/bladder pain syndrome]. Its benefit may arise from patients' empowerment and ability to cope with symptoms."[90]

Indeed, MBSR can help mitigate symptoms of fibromyalgia[91, 92] and urge incontinence.[93]

Another example of a mindfulness-based modality that has been used to reduce chronic pain is loving-kindness, or *metta*, meditation, which cultivates the state of mind known as compassion. For veterans with post-traumatic stress disorder (PTSD), loving-kindness meditation practice is associated with improved positive emotions and might be helpful for reducing stress,[94] and is associated with improved positive emotions in the same population.[95]

In a pilot study by Fox, Flynn, and Allen (2011), mindfulness meditation showed significant improvement in all mindfulness scores for women with chronic pelvic pain.[96] In a different article titled "Experiencing wellness within illness: Exploring a mindfulness-based approach to chronic back pain," mindfulness meditation helped patients with low back pain by "Learning to respond rather than react, and living moment by moment enabled participants to replace a cycle of suffering with one of acceptance. Rather than fearing pain, participants found ways to move through it and live with it."[97] Mindfulness meditation helped the participants identify early warning signs that *precede* a pain flare-up. This helped stop the cycle of projecting past experience of pain onto a fear of future pain and helped them become more flexible in their attitude toward pain. It also reduced self-blame and inner conflict.[98]

McManus (2012) observes that:

> A patient's ability to be aware of the body is necessary for the self-regulation of the nervous system. Many patients have little or no body awareness. Others are afraid to pay attention to their physical experience because of pain. Unable to bring awareness to the body in a skillful manner, they are unable to observe and successfully modulate the stress reaction.[99]

One study concluded that another modality for intervention in patients with pain, mindfulness-based cognitive therapy (MBCT), "can start a process of change in patients with persistent MUS [medically unexplained symptoms]. Awareness and acceptance of painful symptoms and emotions are key factors in this process. Change of unhelpful behavioral patterns and increased self-care and self-compassion can result from this process."[100] This is similar to understanding our *kleshas*, or obstructions to wellness.

Cultivating mindfulness can also be helpful in injury prevention and athletic performance. In the sports setting, a 2018 study screened college athletes for various skills and used mindfulness to improve the mechanics and efficiency of these skills for preseason training and injury prevention.[101] One example of such a skill is the drop vertical jump task, where the subject begins by standing with both legs on a step, and then jumps down onto the floor with both feet. The observer checks the frontal view and films (or observes in real time) the angle of the knees during the landing. Ideally, the angle of the knee in the frontal plane will remain relatively vertical during the landing. Altered frontal plane knee mechanics during dynamic tasks have been often associated with lower extremity injuries such as ACL ligament over-loading.[102] In the 2018 study, "Imposing additional cognitive demands during execution of the drop vertical jump task influenced lower extremity mechanics in a manner that may increase anterior cruciate ligament loading."[103] In other words, being mindful of one's knee angle during landing from a jump may help prevent knee ligament injuries. It certainly helps improve landing mechanics.

The athletic trainer, physical therapist, or strength and conditioning specialist can work with an athlete to (hopefully compassionately) point out the inefficient landing mechanics while encouraging awareness of the athlete's obstruction to wellness, or *klesha*. They would then work on consciously, mindfully, practicing landing mechanics using a new pattern or neuromotor pathway. We practice conscious competence with the goal of the task becoming automatic, so that during a game, the cognitive demands of the sport don't interfere with the landing mechanics. The athlete trains so much that the landing becomes automatic and the athlete is "in the zone," or their body has accomplished "unconscious competence."

Conscious Competence Learning Model

I use the conscious competence learning model[104] to help clients learn new motor patterns. For example, I might say:

> When you first came in to see me, you were not aware that your landing mechanics were less than optimal. We might say that you were not consciously competent, or "unconsciously incompetent" of the best landing strategies when we met. During the evaluation, I compassionately pointed out that you could work on improving your landing mechanics. In that moment, you began to become "consciously incompetent," or aware of the obstructions to changing your knee torque. We quickly moved to practicing "conscious competence" with visual feedback and cues, such as using the mirror, or reviewing a film in slow-motion. The goal now is to practice consciously, so that the new landing skill becomes automatic. Then, you can shift your "brain space" to paying attention to your teammates and the ball on the court. The goal is "unconscious competence," where you don't have to think about the mechanics of landing anymore.

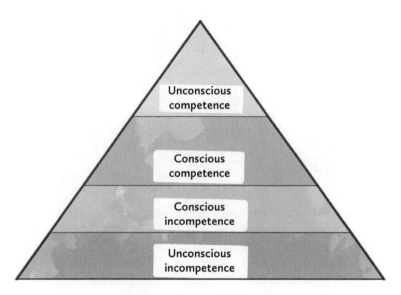

FIGURE 7.1 CONSCIOUS COMPETENCE LEARNING MODEL

I compare the conscious competence theory to learning a new instrument. When we're first tasked with figuring out the fingering on a string or wind instrument, or on a keyboard, it's usually awkward and clumsy. It takes some time to "pluck out" the notes and figure out the fine movement patterns. Integrating these skills requires concentration, or "brain space." Then, slowly, as the fingers "learn" the motor patterns, playing the instrument becomes smoother and up to tempo. By the time a musical performance comes around, the musician has achieved unconscious competence when the composition is memorized. This allows the musician to be able to continue playing while engaging with the audience and other band members, or even singing at the same time. The conscious competence theory is useful clinical reasoning for "buying into" mindfulness practice in the rehabilitation of movement. In reality, how we teach clients depends a lot on the practitioner's experience. It's recommended that "Prior to introducing mindfulness to patients, pain professionals need personal experience practicing mindfulness meditation and integrating mindfulness into daily life."[105]

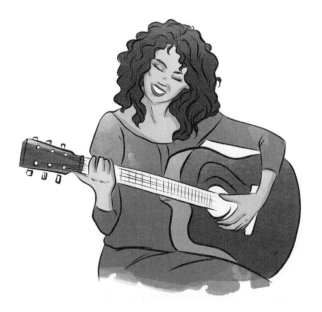

FIGURE 7.2 MINDFULNESS

Let's not conflate learning new movement patterns consciously and mindfully with pain treatment. "Mindfulness Based Stress Reduction (MBSR) therapy is a meditation therapy...originally designed for stress management,"[106] and may be an effective treatment option for patients with chronic low back pain,[107] but it is complicated, and pain is multifactorial. MBSR includes yoga; it is not just a meditation practice. In a study attempting to correlate mindfulness with pain reduction, "Higher pain tolerance through meditation could not be confirmed... We surmise that mindfulness may have the potential to reduce pain, but may not do so 'automatically,' as long as the use of this skill and expected outcomes are not trained simultaneously."[108] The goal is not just about eliminating pain, but *coping with the pain*, understanding its personal, individual sources, and working toward calming our responses to the perception of pain.

Cultivating mindfulness takes practice and time. It is just one of the tools already included in the yoga therapy toolbox to help alleviate individual suffering. Just as it is impossible to separate the layers of health, we cannot tease out all the factors of yoga and yoga therapy that will help alleviate pain and suffering. Yoga therapy works through many mechanisms of the body, mind, and spirit. Mindfulness is included in the list of treatment suggestions to integrate behavioral and psychosocial approaches into physical therapy for patients with chronic pain. (Other suggestions include pain education, diaphragmatic breathing, relaxation techniques, sleep hygiene, and other cognitive and operant restructuring techniques.)[109]

Yoga therapy inherently addresses and includes these treatments in its practice and philosophies. Sullivan et al. propose that an "individual's transformation in the experience of illness, pain, or disability... occurs through facilitating a reharmonization of body, mind, and environment toward the experience of eudaimonic well-being."[110] Eudaimonia, an ancient Greek concept "often defined as a life well-lived or well-intentioned," blends seamlessly with the practice of yoga, or "a well-lived life of fulfilled meaning and purpose."[111]

This includes living with less suffering and pain.

Pain Science

Acute pain caused by tissue damage is a condition that is easy for most people to intuitively understand because most of us have experienced this type of pain at various times in our lives. *Chronic* pain is different and not as easily understood. Moreover, it is often the case that imaging studies do not correlate with the experience of subjective pain reports.[112, 113, 114, 115] In other words, there are far too many cases where the imaging shows tissue damage without subjective reports of pain, and vice versa. Emerging medical guidelines "'strongly' discourage the use of MRI [magnetic resonance imaging] and X-ray in diagnosing low back pain, because they produce so many false alarms."[116] And patients with radiating leg pain who were shown to have the presence of nerve root compression and extrusion of a herniated disc on an MRI reported "less leg pain during 1-year follow-up, irrespective of a surgical or conservative treatment."[117]

In other words, "MRI findings seem not to be helpful in determining which patients might fare better with early surgery compared with a strategy of prolonged conservative care."[118] I see this in my practice, too. Most of the time, clients who learn to manage the ups and downs of their pain psychologically and learn physically how to control their spinal stability in their daily life and activities tend to fare well without surgery. And those who do end up requiring surgery tend to have easier recoveries if they have built up their sustainable core resilience before surgery.

We all relate to pain differently. One of my favorite extreme examples of this is told by psychoneurobiologist Rachel Zoffness in her blog post "A tale of two nails." For an unforgettable X-ray image, check out this post! She reminds us that pain is not a purely biological process. "Thoughts, beliefs, perceptions, emotions, past experiences, context, and input from your body all affect our experience of pain… And not just some of the time, but all of the time, always."[119] To demonstrate this point, she relates the example of a man with a nail stuck in his boot (he thought it was penetrating his foot, but it wasn't) and who was in agonizing pain, contrasted with another man who didn't even realize that a nail had been pierced through his head for six days! She reminds us that "Pain is never purely biological, due exclusively to issues like tissue damage and anatomical dysfunction. It is also emotional, social and cognitive, constantly influenced by thoughts, perceptions, emotions, and context."[120] In other words, pain is multifactorial—it is psychological and social, too! We can best address pain with the biopsychosocial-spiritual (BPSS) approach.

Research shows that using a neuroplasticity explanation, rather than a traditional biomechanical explanation, to educate participants with chronic low back pain, results in "a measurable difference in SLR [straight leg raise] in patients with CLBP [chronic low back pain] when receiving manual therapy."[121] Furthermore, the randomized clinical trial "Effect of Pain Reprocessing Therapy vs Placebo and Usual Care for Patients with Chronic Back Pain" concludes, "Psychological treatment centered on changing patients' beliefs about the causes and threat value of pain may provide substantial and durable pain relief for people with chronic back pain."[122] Pain is a sensation that is interpreted in the brain,[123] and yoga practice and philosophy can help us understand the causes of our pain or suffering.

In yoga philosophy, another concept closely related to ignorance or one of the *kleshas*, *avidya*, is that of *duhkha*. Desikachar notes that "Sometimes terms such as 'suffering,' 'troubles,' or 'sickness' are used to explain the meaning of duhkha, but it is best described as a feeling of being restricted. Duhkha is a quality of mind that gives us the feeling of being squeezed."[124] It is not the same as physical pain. "Duhkha is nothing but a certain state of mind in which we experience a limitation of our possibilities to act and understand."[125] Conversely, "When we feel a sense of lightness and openness within, then we are experiencing the opposite of duhkha, a state that is called sukha," literally, a good space.[126] This is where yoga comes in as a healing modality. "We all have the goal of eliminating duhkha... That is what yoga tries to achieve,"[127] Desikachar states.

The second chapter of Patanjali's *Yoga Sutra* (2:15) says, "To one of discrimination, everything is painful..."[128] Satchidanada teaches us that if we don't have the experience of gaining something that is desired, then we won't fear losing it. But once we have a pleasurable experience, we have the memory and "the resulting impressions left in the mind to create renewed cravings; and the constant conflict among the three gunas, which control the mind."[129]

Our minds are always in flux and, with practice, one can choose to respond to their thoughts of fear, anxiety, and pain (whether physical or mental) with more grace and ease. When the health care provider is aware of these constant mental fluctuations in their clients, and ideally has some experience in responding kindly to such thoughts arising within themselves, it is easier to guide others.

Compassionate Health Care

According to O'Keeffe (2016), "A mix of interpersonal, clinical, and organizational factors are perceived to influence patient-therapist interactions, although research is needed to identify which of these factors actually influence patient-therapist interactions. Physical therapists' awareness of these factors could enhance patient interactions and treatment outcomes."[130] For low back pain, "identification of areas of convergence and divergence of approaches is designed to clarify the key aspects of each approach and thereby serve as a guide for the clinician and to provide a platform for considering a hybrid approach tailored to the individual patient."[131] We might be more successful when we meet the client where they are and get a sense of their awareness, eudaimonia, and interoception, to help them rehabilitate mindfully. "Yoga aims to facilitate the emergence of qualities such as eudaimonia by strengthening the experience of *sattva.*"[132]

Recall that in Sullivan et al.'s (2018) article "Yoga therapy and polyvagal theory,"[133] the authors relate three neural platforms discussed in polyvagal theory with the three *gunas*, or qualities of nature. The three polyvagal neural platforms—the ventral vagal complex (VVC), the sympathetic nervous system (SNS), and the dorsal vagal complex (DVC)—are compared to the behaviors of healthy social engagement, defensive strategy of mobilization (fight or flight), and defensive strategy of immobilization (freeze) respectively.

Guna	Sattva	Rajas	Tamas
Vagal state	Homeostasis	Fight/flight	Freeze
Neural platform	Ventral vagal complex (VVC)	Sympathetic nervous system (SNS)	Dorsal vagal complex (DVC)
Behavior	Social engagement	Defensive strategy of mobilization	Defensive strategy of immobilization

FIGURE 7.3 THE *GUNAS*

As Desikachar explains, "Every action that stems from avidyā always leads to one or another form of duḥkha."[134] Furthermore, to understand *duhkha*, we must understand the three qualities of mind described by yoga—*tamas, rajas*, and *sattva*.[135] Together these three qualities are known as the *gunas*, which is Sanskrit for strands or qualities. In yoga anatomy, there is an in-between layer that is neither solely physical nor solely spiritual, called the subtle body. Western scientists have started to explore the subtle body concept in research on meditation.[136] I like to think of the non-dualistic, in-between layers as the energetic body.

In yoga philosophy one goal is to cultivate a state of balance, or *sattva*, in which our nervous system is in homeostasis and we are socially engaged. However, our physiological energies are always in flux, and the states of defense (mobilization or immobilization) are always present under the surface to some degree. Safely practicing and mindfully experiencing states of fight, flight, or freeze strengthens our resilience (physically and mentally). Yoga helps us cultivate resilience "by strengthening the experience of sattva and VVC as well as developing facility in moving between *gunas* and neural platforms and changing the relationship and response to the inherent changing nature of the body, mind and environment reflected in *gunas* and neural platforms."[137]

CULTIVATING A SUSTAINABLE CORE

In yoga therapy and yoga philosophy it is considered vital to distinguish between those aspects of experience that are constantly changing and those that are unchanging and immutable. Prakriti is the term that encompasses all malleable and fluctuating components of the body, mind and environment. Purusha represents an aspect of the unchanging experience of awareness through which unwavering equanimity arises.[138] "Within Prakriti, resilience is represented by the capacity to recognize and shift states, as well as changing the relationship to the fluctuations of the *gunas* (rajas/tamas/sattva) and neural platforms (sympathetic nervous system (SNS)/dorsal vagal complex (DVC)/ventral vagal complex (VVC))."[139]

So, in the studio, once clients begin to get a grasp on their bony alignment and the muscle contraction patterns and breathing habits which help them stay centered, I invite them to become aware, or mindful, that movement patterns, just like thoughts, are constantly in flux. Yoga therapy rehabilitation practice includes recognizing the habits which help keep us centered (versus those which don't serve us) and then actively practicing the positions and postures which cultivate centered resilience and strengthen the experience of peace, social engagement, and homeostasis, or *sattva*. Their homework includes not beating themselves up if they find themselves in a painful position. Instead, the practice is to change their posture immediately to a more comfortable position, take a deep breath, and carry on. Eventually, this comfortable mindfulness becomes automatic, or unconsciously competent, and the goal of attaining less suffering is possible.

8

THE ENERGETIC CORE

Gunas

In Yoga philosophy the *gunas* are the energetic forces that weave together to form the universe and everything in it.[1] As noted in the previous chapter, there are three *gunas*, each with their own unique attributes: *tamas* (stability), *rajas* (activity), and *sattva* (consciousness). We possess various portions of all these qualities at any given time. "The recognition of an underlying abiding equanimity amidst the fluctuating stimuli of the body, mind, and world can create a broadening of the field of attention and a larger context for the experience of, and reaction to, sensation."[2]

Practicing yoga invites us to become more aware of our ever-changing subtle energies within the context of our everyday life. Yoga anatomy and physiology includes the idea of subtle energy or life force. This life force, compared to *chi* or *qi* in Traditional Chinese Medicine (TCM), is called *Prana* in yoga. I don't intend to completely explain the yoga philosophy of subtle energy; that is not the scope of this text. However, I do hope to provide enough information to pique your interest and introduce the surface of complex deep concepts. I hope that by reading about these subtle energies, you might be curious about them and perhaps become inquisitive about how your own body feels when it is digesting food or thoughts.

Prana

Yoga instructor and writer Rolf Sovik notes, "Like the changing designs of a kaleidoscope, patterns of energy within the body/mind are continually refashioning themselves… Every individual pattern of energy is a configuration of five primary energy functions, called the five forces of Prana."[3] *Prana*, with a capital P, is understood as a universal energy or life force, which flows in currents in and around the body. Prana is *not* our breath. The concept of *Prana* as a life force can be thought of as an energy being "carried" into the body on the breath. This energy "rides" within the oxygen molecules as it circulates through the body. We might think of the energy *charge* carried on the molecule as an example of *Prana*. Bhavanani and Ramanathan observe that when our *Prana* is flowing freely and harmoniously, we are in a healthy state. Health is also further understood as harmonious balance of *prana vayus* (major physiological energy) and *upana prana vayus* (minor energies of physiological function), coupled with stability of *nadis* (subtle energy channels) and harmonious flow of energy through all *chakras*.[4]

Nadis

Prana, the subtle flow of vibration, sometimes called the "breath of life," travels through the body on channels or energetic vessels called the *nadis*.[5] There are thousands of *nadis*, which "are described as thin strand like threads, similar to those of the lotus stem, which emanate from the spinal column."[6] *Nadis* overlap with, and can be compared to, the acupressure meridians. The three main, and most important, *nadis* are the three central ones: the *susumna, ida,* and *pingala nadis*.

The *susumna nadi*, the *nadi* of fire, is the main channel for the flow of nervous energy, and it is vertical and centrally situated inside the spinal column. "In recent times the *nadi* system has been associated with the nervous system."[7] The human body can be thought of as a miniature universe. The Sanskrit syllable *ha* means sun and *tha* means moon. Together, we get the word *hatha*, or force. The lunar energy is said to flow in the *ida nadi*, which begins in the left nostril. The solar energy flows in the *pingala nadi*, which starts from the right nostril. Both energies move down to the base of the spine. These three central energy channels weave and intersect with themselves at certain points in our central midline. Those of us in the Western medical field might recognize this image as the caduceus, or the symbol associated with medicine. The *nadis* intersect at, and energetically feed, the *chakras*, or energy centers, in the subtle body.

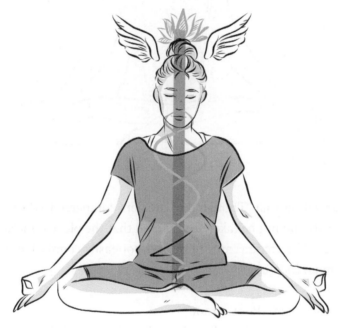

FIGURE 8.1 THE *NADIS*

Chakras

B. K. S. Iyengar, an Indian teacher of yoga and author, explains that "The chakras are the regions situated within the spinal column where the nādis cross each other."[8] The seven (main) *chakras* are "energy vortexes that govern our physical, emotional, mental, spiritual well-being."[9] In TCM, all the acupressure meridians run through the *chakra* centers and most of the pressure points correspond to the characteristics of the nearest *chakra*.[10] "From a neuro-physiological perspective, the chakras are represented as nerve plexuses from the spinal column and endocrine glands that connect with the internal organs."[11]

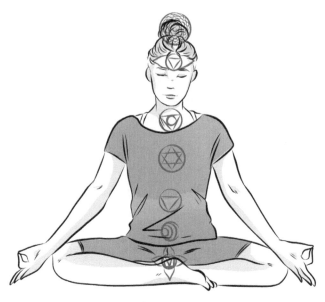

FIGURE 8.2 THE *CHAKRAS*

Iyengar tells us that "Though they are here compared to the various plexi, it should not be taken for granted that the plexi alone are the chakras... The chakras are subtle and not easily cognisable."[12] The seven main *chakras* are:

- *muladhara* (Root): "root"
- *svadhisthana* (Sacral): "where the self is established"
- *manipura* (Solar Plexus): "jewel city"
- *anahata* (Heart): "un-struck"
- *vishuddha* (Throat): "purist"
- *ajna* (Third Eye/Brow): "command center"
- *sahasrara* (Crown): "thousand-petaled lotus."

These *nadi* junctions, the *chakras*, regulate the body mechanism like fly-wheels regulate an engine. According to the Tantric texts the object of *pranayama* is to arouse the divine cosmic force in our bodies. Like a snake or caduceus, these energies are symbolized "as a coiled and sleeping serpent lying dormant in the lowest nerve centre at the base of the spinal column, the Mūlādhāra [root] Chakra."[13]

According to hatha and tantric yoga lineages, "This latent energy has to be aroused and made to go up the spinal column piercing the chakras up to the Sahasrāra (the thousand-petalled lotus in the head, the network of nerves in the brain) and there to unite with the Supreme Soul."[14] When this happens, we temporarily reach *samadhi*, or Bliss, or Union with the Divine. Again, this state is temporary. While it might be a goal to attain such bliss, we cannot live our day-to-day lives in heavenly ecstasy. Our energies, or *prana*, are constantly shifting between states of bliss, action, and rest.

Vayus

Prana can be divided into many parts, but there are five main *vayus*, or *pancha pranas*, that are the most important for yoga practitioners to understand. The five *vayus* are: *apana vayu, prana vayu, samana vayu, udana vayu*, and *vyana vayu*.[15] The two *vayus* that are usually easiest to grasp are *prana vayu* and *apana vayu*. Yoga instructor and author Timothy Burgin states that "Once you connect with the subtle energies of these two Vayus it will be easier to work with the others."[16]

Burgin explains how *prana-vayu* or acquisition of energy "is situated in the heart, and its energy pervades the chest region. Prana-Vayu translates as 'forward-moving air,' and its flow is inwards and upward."[17] *Prana vayu* energy circulates all around the body from the heart. Clinical psychologist and yoga instructor Rolf Sovik writes: "The acquisition of energy, or prana [vayu], is characterized as an upward-moving process ('filling-up') and it is associated with the chest and throat.[18] Burgin concurs and adds that *prana-vayu* "nourishes the brain and the eyes and governs the intake of reception of all things: food, air, senses, and thoughts. This *vayu* is the fundamental energy in the body and directs and feeds into the four other *Vayus*.[19] One can also imagine this energy flowing from the belly to the third eye, while residing in the thorax. This flow can be sealed or controlled with a throat lock, or *jalandhara bandha*. Its associated chakras and elements are Anahata (heart) and air.[20] When someone swells up with emotion and has a lump in their throat, I imagine this is *prana vayu* expanding from the belly and heart, unconsciously halted or sealed with the vocal folds.

Apana vayu, or elimination, "is symbolized as a downward-moving process ('emptying out') and is associated with the lower abdomen and pelvic floor. It governs such functions as urination, defecation, and menses."[21] This energy can be stopped or controlled with the practice of *mula bandha*, or root lock, which is an advanced, energetic version of a pelvic floor muscle contraction, to be discussed soon. *Apana vayu* translates as "the air that moves away," and its flow is downward and out. Its energy nourishes the organs of digestion, reproduction, and elimination. Its expression is steadiness, and its associated *chakras* and elements are *muladhara* (root) and earth.[22]

Samana vayu is centered at the navel region (the solar plexus) of the abdomen and governs the absorption of energy.[23, 24] "The location of Samana Vayu is especially important because it rests in the middle ground between prana vayu in the chest and apana vayu in the pelvic floor." We can seal this energy with *uddiyana bandha*, or abdominal lock. *Samana vayu* translates to "the balancing air,"[25] and its flow moves from the periphery of the body to the center. "From this hub energy radiates outward to the rest of the body in channels called nadis."[26] Its associated *chakras* and elements are *manipura* (solar plexus) and fire.[27] I think of *samana vayu* as our gut energy.

Udana vayu "is situated in the throat, and it has a circular flow around the neck and head."[28] *Udana vayu* "translates to 'that which carries upward,' and its flow moves up from the heart to the head, five senses and brain."[29] Its energy passes through the pharynx and helps maintain upright posture and governs speech, self-expression, and growth. This *vayu*'s action is metabolization, its expression is verbal, and its associated *chakras* and elements are *vishuddha* (throat), *anja* (third eye) and ether.[30] Just like the upward flow of *prana vayu*, we can also pause *udana vayu* energy with a throat lock or *jalandhara bandha*.

Vyana vayu is associated with circulation and can be linked with the heart and lungs. *Vyana vayu* "is situated in the heart and lungs and flows throughout the entire body. Vyana-vayu translates as 'outward-moving air,' and its flow moves from the center of the body to the periphery."[31] Its expression is alignment, and its associated *chakras* and elements are *svadisthana* (sacral) and water. "The activities of prana, apana, and samana, along with the other two functions of Prana (vyana and udana – the forces involved in the distribution of energy within the body/mind and in certain special functions such as speech), comprise one layer in the pattern of human energy."[32]

There are multiple layers of energy assimilating our food and thoughts, oscillating and balancing with each other consistently throughout the day and night. Whether we are aware of them or not, yogis are showing us that we can learn how to control and redirect them with energetic and muscular contractions.

Simply being curious or open-minded about the idea that these subtle energies might exist, let alone that we can observe, feel, and redirect them, is my suggestion. The awareness that there might be an entire cosmos of action inside our bodies fascinates me. I love knowing that there is more going on inside the body than we can observe with the naked eye.

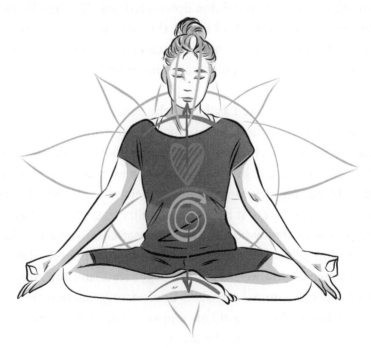

FIGURE 8.3 THE *VAYUS*

Remember, we cannot separate the energetic body from the physical body. Deeper studies and practice of yoga reveals that when we engage the pelvic floor muscles (PFM) or "seal off and control the anatomical perineum – the base of the pelvis…[we] cultivate…abdomino-pelvic energy."[33] This energy and strength translates up through the core cylinder. For example, while singing, the PFM "establish a foundation for creating an intensely lyric sound… [F]or singers and public speakers who are engaging an audience, a tripartite muscular effort within the torso is apparent."[34] The PFM, transverse abdominis muscle (TVA), and respiratory diaphragm muscle (RD) "act together to oversee a whole-body regulation of the passage of air past the vocal cords in the larynx."[35]

In *The Heart of Yoga*, T. K. V. Desikachar discusses how *pranayama* helps to reduce waste matter in the body by directing *agni*, the fire of life.[36] This flame is said to reside in the navel, between the *prana vayu* and *apana vayu*. "The flame itself is constantly changing direction: on inhalation the breath moves toward the belly, causing a draft that directs the flame downward, just like in a fireplace; during exhalation the draft moves the flame in the opposite direction,"[37] burning off waste matter. A complete exhalation is needed to rid the body of its rubbish and maintain health. *Bandhas* can intensify this practice.

"Roughly translated as 'locks,' the *bandhas* are presented as a series of internal hydraulics by which physical and psychic energies may be forcefully channeled within the body."[38] Remember that the physical energies in the abdomen behave according to the laws of hydraulic physics, and the thorax behaves according to pneumatic physics. "Were it not for our ability to supplement skeletal support with the hydraulic and pneumatic pressures within the abdomino-pelvic and thoracic cavities, the intervertebral discs in the lumbar region would quickly degenerate and rupture."[39] We need intra-abdominal pressure. Coulter suggests that we can do this with or without the aid of compressed air in the chest in three ways: (1) we can hold our breath and *close* the glottis (mostly recommended for emergencies or trained situations), (2) we can keep the glottis open and use the PFM, TVA, and RD to modulate the pressures as we move through space (preferred), and (3) the most natural way, which is to mix the two strategies.[40] We can practice isolating muscles to improve their responsiveness, but that is just the foundation. Once we are able to control the individual sections of the body symphony, we can put them together for efficient movement strategies.

With these energetics in mind, let's dive a little deeper into the three diaphragms individually. In yoga, there are more advanced practices to consciously activate and strengthen the diaphragm muscles. As the intensity and load against pressure increases, so do the risks of injury if one does not build the reliance gradually over time. In other words, up until now in this book, I have been conscious about offering gentle, light, soft practices that should be accessible to most people. To build resilience and strength, we need to *gradually and methodically* introduce challenge, load, and/ or pressure.

At the risk of over-cautioning the reader, if you decide to explore energy-locking exercises, please seek individual guidance from an experienced yoga teacher or therapist. It is contraindicated to perform *bandhas* if you have any of the following conditions: high or low blood pressure, hernias, ulcers in the stomach or intestines, or if you have or have recently had any other abdominal illness or trauma, glaucoma, or heart disease.[41] Most yoga traditions advise against this practice or any breath retention during menses or pregnancy.[42] It's best to practice on an empty stomach, and before beginning, to evacuate the bladder and bowels.[43] As we move away from the material, concrete ideas of bones, structure, and muscles, and how they mechanically work together to breathe, I invite you to consider the more subtle and energetic aspects of exercise and yoga.

"When prāṇa is made to flow in the yogi's body by the practice of prāṇāyāma," Iyengar says, "it is equally necessary for him to employ bandhas to prevent the dissipation of energy and to carry it to the right quarters without causing damage elsewhere."[44]

Mudras and *Bandhas*

"*Mudra*" means "seal."[45] In yoga, *mudras* are gestures, usually per-formed with the hands and fingers, used in conjunction with *pran-ayama* to stimulate different parts of the body to affect the flow of *prana*.[46] "In texts such as the *Hatha-Yoga-Pradipika* it is suggested that certain practices that focus the mind can center the prana. These are termed mudras."[47] Common forms of mudras are certain hand postures, like *anjali* mudra where the palms are placed together like a lotus flower, similar to the "prayer position" or gesture where one places their palms together, fingers pointed up, and the thumbs placed near the heart or forehead. This *mudra* is often used in the Sanskrit greeting of "namaste," or at the end of a yoga class to seal the intention of a practice. Another common hand gesture is the *gyan mudra*—the gesture of knowledge or wisdom where we place the tip of the thumb to the tip of the index finger. Often people use this *mudra* while seated cross-legged for an inwardly focused meditation. Other *mudras* from the sacred texts include headstand, shoulder-stand, and *shan mukhi* mudra, where we close the eyes, ears, and mouth with our fingers and thumbs. Mohan and Mohan (2004) teach us that "The practice of mudras helps to prevent the scattering of prana and thus aids in achieving focus of the mind."[48] Vernikos et al. (2012) explore the neurological effects of *mudras*, suggesting that *mudras* "act as switches for neuro-physical transmission pathways directing the flow of the '*prāna-shakti*,' or 'life energy,' to diseased organs in order to heal them."[49]

In several ancient yoga texts, "Bandhas are also grouped with mudras, as they serve the same purpose."[50] Both *mudras* and *band-has* can be used to redirect *prana*. In Sanskrit, "The word *bandha* means 'to bind, or tie together, to close.' In the way it is used in yoga, *bandha* also means 'to lock.'"[51] In his book *Light on Yoga*, Iyengar states, "*Bandha* means bondage, joining together, fettering, or catching hold of. It is also a posture in which certain organs or parts of the body are contracted and controlled."[52] "Without the *bandhas*, prāṇa is lethal."[53]

"*Bandhas* include certain physical practices involving muscular contractions, designed to block off or seal off certain areas of the body and thus redirect the flow of *prana*."[54] The practice of "binding" concentrates or "locks" energy into focused areas of the body.[55] "An important use of the *bandhas* is to enhance the function of *agni*, or digestive energy. This happens more as a result of appropriate breathing than from bodywork."[56] In other words, *bandhas* are not practiced in isolation. Three important *bandhas* used in *pranayama* practice are *mula bandha* in the pelvis, *uddiyana bandha* in the abdomen, and *jalandhara bandha* in the throat.

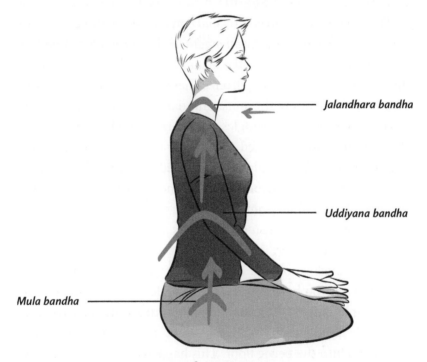

FIGURE 8.4 THE *BANDHAS*

Iyengar warns that "There is a grave danger in attempting to learn [Uddiyana and Mula] Bandhas by oneself, without the personal supervision of an experienced Guru or teacher."[57] For this reason, please note that the images we include to illustrate the location of the three common *bandhas* are *not* the traditional way to practice

them—they are modified toward a neutral spine zone as an introduction for beginners as a gateway to explore the subtle energetics
of yoga.

Mula bandha practice involves contraction of the pelvic floor
and lower abdomen muscles below the navel. Recall that when we
perform a Kegel, the lower TVA contracts naturally with the PFM.
"Extended exhalation involves the contraction of the abdominal
muscles and thus performing *mula bandha* in suspension after exhalation allows one to use the natural link between muscular work and
the breathing process."[58] Note the inclusion of a complete exhalation.

The *pelvic* diaphragm is activated consciously by three isometric
practices: *vajroli mudra*, *ashwini mudra*, and *mula bandha*. Anatomi-
cally, the perineum refers to the diamond-shaped area between the
anus and genitals, extending from either the vaginal opening to the
anus or the scrotum to the anus. This diamond can be divided into
posterior and anterior triangles. The perineal body is an irregular
fibro-muscular mass, located at the central point of the perineum.
The anterior half of the diamond is called the urogenital triangle,
while the posterior portion is termed the posterior anal triangle.
Vajroli mudra is a light, isometric closure of the urethral opening in
the urogenital triangle. *Ashwini mudra* is a conscious closure of the
external anal sphincter.

Ashwini means horse or mare, and as we have stated, a *mudra*
is a gesture. If you have ever seen a horse defecate, you might note
that the anus bulges a little and, right after the contents of the anus
are expelled, the muscles around it "wink" and the anus reflexively
retracts up into the pelvic floor. This happens in humans, too. We
reflexively pull our posterior pelvic floor from moment to moment
throughout our day. *Ashwini mudra* is the practice of contracting and
releasing the posterior triangle of the pelvic floor and traditionally
includes recruitment of the gluteal muscles, deep/posterior pelvic
diaphragm, and sphincter. The position of the feet and hips affects
the recruitment of the pelvic floor muscles.[59] It is easier to isolate the
posterior triangle and relax the anterior portion when our heels and
toes are together, with our hips externally rotated, and the spine is

in slight extension (and it is more difficult with our toes out, hips abducted, and spine flexed, such as in a standing wide angle forward fold).[60] This is useful when exploring our own awareness of the diaphragms in the body. *Ashwini mudra* is a sharper, more forceful contraction of the posterior triangle of the pelvic floor than *mula bandha*, which is an upward/vertical lifting of the (perineal) body, or the central fascial point. *Mula bandha* is said to seal or stop the downward, digestive energy of flow in the body, called *apana vayu*.

While *mula bandha* in the pelvic floor energetically seals the bottom of the core cylinder, *jalandhara bandha* stops the upward flow of *prana* at the top of the cylinder in the throat. The throat lock seals the naturally occurring upward *prana vayu* and *udana vayu* energies in the body that are associated with the intake and circulation of air, water, and food. The traditional throat seal involves rounding the upper back and slightly hyperextending the neck so that the chin is touching the chest. Obviously, this requires a lot of flexibility and strength in the neck and back. For this reason, I am sticking to a theoretical discussion of the energy locks for this text.

Uddiyana bandha pauses the absorption of energy in the solar plexus, and its practice is related to *mula bandha*. *Uddiyana bandha* involves contraction of the upper abdominal muscles, drawing the navel upward and inward. "When done properly, *jalandhara-bandha* helps in doing mula-bandha."[61] Mohan and Mohan (2004) remind us that the breath is a part of bandha practice and "lengthening and controlling the breath in asana practice is essential before attempting to do *jalandhara-bandha*."[62] They further caution that *uddiyana bandha* and *mula bandha* "are not to be attempted on inhalation and in backbends. They should be done after exhalation, slowly, with awareness, and with *jalandhara bandha*."[63] Once the throat and pelvis lock are accomplished in the practice of *pranayama*, "they are to be maintained throughout while *uddiyana bandha* is to be done on suspension after exhalation and released before inhalation."[64] Again, I introduce this as an academic exercise for the reader to contemplate. The purpose of the *bandhas* "is to prevent the prana from moving upward and the apana from moving downward so that both are retained."[65] There is a lot going on in our body beneath our consciousness and, with practice and guided supervision, one can not only learn how to recognize the subtle shifts in energy, but to direct and manipulate it at will. This is one of the superpowers of yoga.

Modified *Maha Mudra*

Iyengar explains that *maha* means great or noble.[66] *Mudra* also means shutting, closing, or sealing. The advanced and extreme seated yoga posture named *maha mudra* closes the apertures at the top and bottom of the trunk and are held fast and sealed. Recall from Chapter 5, The Muscular Core, that when the sustainable core muscles are engaged in neutral spine, the three diaphragms are parallel, and a unique action emerges: axial extension. The "seated posture named mahamudra...adds a twisting action to axial extension. It is considered a supreme accomplishment to do this practice with all three bandhas executed correctly, because it represents a complete merging of asana and pranayama practice."[67]

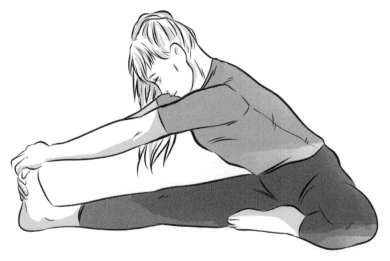

FIGURE 8.5 MODIFIED *MAHA BANDHA*

Reminder: the images we chose to introduce *maha mudra* and the *bandhas* are not the traditional way to practice the poses—they are modified as an introduction for beginners as a gateway to gently explore the subtle energetics of yoga. Desikachar suggests that "We should begin practicing the bandhas in simple āsanas so that the body can get used to them."[68] He recommends that we practice the bandhas first in the supine position with our arms overhead, then in downward-facing dog or other inversions, and eventually in sitting positions like *mahamudra* prior to combining them with breathing practices. He reminds us that the *bandhas* intensify the cleansing effect of *pranayama* with *agni*, our digestive, life fire. The chin-lock positions the trunk in such a way that "the spine is held erect. This makes it easier for the prana to move the flame towards the rubbish that needs burning."[69] The upward-abdominal lock "then raises the rubbish up toward the flame, and mūla bandha helps us leave it there long enough for the rubbish to be burned."[70]

The traditional version of *maha mudra* is a rigorous pose involving the combination of the three *bandhas* while seated in a wide-angle pose with one knee bent (half knee to nose pose) and the heel of the bent leg contacting the perineum. In a traditional chin lock, the neck is flexed and retracted to the point where the chin rests on the hollow between the collarbones just above the sternum (not shown). The seals are engaged and the breath held for an instructed amount of time that is supervised by an experienced teacher. This *asana* is known to mobilize the abdominal organs and is said to cure indigestion, perhaps because it flips and stretches the three diaphragm muscles physically (recall that the esophagus pierces directly through the RDM) while simultaneously halting the breath and the subtle body's energy flow, which includes the energy of circulation and digestion (in light of the *vayus*). Iyengar tells us that "This Mahāmudrā destroys death and many other pains."[71] Doesn't that sound like a nice long-term goal to strive for?

In conclusion, if we simply entertain the idea that subtle energies exist and that with attention and practice one can shift them at will, why wouldn't we want to tap into that to alleviate our suffering? We can use *asana*, or physical postures, as a window into our internal universe. We can investigate what happens when we safely place ourselves in awkward or unstable positions. How does our body respond?

We can explore questions on the mat such as: What are the three diaphragms doing to support our dynamic trunk stability? Is our physical body resilient, flexible, graceful, humble, controlled, smooth? What about our emotional or energetic body? Or do we recruit our superficial, emergency core muscles, increase our intra-abdominal pressure, and hold our breath in unstable situations? When teaching clients new movement patterns, I ask them to observe their breath. I suggest that if they are holding their breath, they might have gone past their "edge." I invite them to play with this "edge" of control and ease to investigate patterns, perceived or real limitations, and possibilities for movement and transformation.

That said, breath holding for extreme weightlifting is a safe strategy, when one gradually builds up strength and tissue integrity in a graded, progressive, manner. But in the case of general physical therapy, yoga, and rehabilitation, I recommend avoiding breath holding as an everyday stability strategy. Or at the very least, I suggest we notice and become aware of the times we use that strategy. Most importantly, can we slow down, back up, and redo the movement mindfully coordinated with the breath? If not, let's be curious and safely explore the barriers.

When assessing clients for movement efficiency, or a sustainable core, I watch their chosen movement or posture related to their goals and observe five things:

1. Are they able to center their range of motion and find axial extension? Are they avoiding extreme spinal end-ranges of motion?
2. Are they controlling their movement with their sustainable core muscles? Or are they recruiting their emergency breathing muscles, and/or using increased intra-abdominal pressure, as a central stability strategy?
3. Are they breathing smoothly through the desired task? Or are they holding their breath for a core stability strategy?

4. Are they moving with self-awareness and grace? Or do their movements look awkward or out of control?

5. Are they open-minded to understanding that they are capable of changing their movement and thought patterns to create more resilience and less suffering? Or are they just going through the motions because a professional is telling them to?

In other words, are they: aware of their alignment, using efficient core muscle strategies, and breathing mindfully with their movement? If so, are they carefully exploring new or previously scary movements, while listening to the signals and sensations which arise, and are constantly fluctuating in their body? Is there clear bottom-up signal reception from their body to their brain? Does their mind interpret their sensations in a healthy way? Then, are they open to changing their habitual responses or old ways of posturing throughout their day? Are they interested in turning these novel movements or habits into daily homework and are they committed to practicing their new movement patterns? Are they open to the idea that their old compensatory strategies might be related to their complaints or suffering?

If they are seeking physical or yoga therapy because they have pain during a certain movement or activity, such as reaching their arms overhead, I observe them performing the activity. In this case, is the client shrugging (elevating) their shoulder/scapula to extreme end-range and holding their breath while they reach to the top shelf for a teacup? What happens if they readjust their posture toward a neutral spine zone as they approach the cupboard? Could they readjust their trunk to achieve more axial extension? If so, can they lift their arm and flex their shoulder with good co-contraction of the "wings" (scapular stabilizers) and transverse abdominis muscle? What if they attempt to coordinate their movement with their breath? Does it change their symptom if they exhale as they elevate their arm? Conversely, what if they *inhale* smoothly while their hand floats up to the cup? If I find they indeed feel better with a slight adjustment to one of these aspects, I suggest that the next time they are moving about in their day and feel their symptom, they might stop, readjust their position toward the task, and redo the action mindfully with less suffering.

I invite them to explore practicing the activity again in a pain-free, perhaps smaller/shorter range of motion, or symptom-reducing manner, which is a new bottom-up signal from the body to the brain. I suggest that they try a new movement pattern when they are not pressed for time. For example, I recommend they pause and think about reaching for a cup before moving, and then execute the movement slowly and mindfully, while consciously breathing with the movement.

If we cannot find a modified movement that reduces symptoms, more exploration is necessary (tests, measures, referrals). The more we practice the pain-free pattern consciously, with less suffering, the more likely it is that we will be able to attain unconscious competence.

Another way to think about it is as if we are learning a new language, or a new way of communicating between the body and the brain. The more we practice novel movements that cause less suffering, the sooner the "pre-flex" winking of the PF, TVA, and wings get "back online," and eventually it happens automatically (unconscious competence). But if we ignore the symptoms and push through our end-ranges against high loads that we have not gradually trained for, we miss the warning signals that our body is capable of subtly producing. When we ignore our symptoms and push through them, the body doesn't "know" that there isn't a life-or-death situation. It might respond as if in an emergency, where the brain overrides the symptoms and completes the task even if tissue rupturing is felt or heard. This is not a healthy "mind over matter" capability. It is an unhealthy, and unfortunately all too common, top-down strategy to use in our everyday life to "just get through." Instead, I advise clients to relearn the task with a smaller range of motion and decreased load until they restore their sequence and timing of the PFM, TVA, and "wings." Once they restore the sequence and timing of the sustainable core muscles with their breath, then we can add more load and increase the ranges of motion gradually toward their goals.

To recap, the mechanics of the five components of building a sustainable core are:

- finding your center
- coordinating the efficient core muscles
- synchronizing the core muscles with the breath
- mindfulness of movement and postures
- practicing novel ways of being within your body and mind to alleviate suffering.

The fifth step to cultivating a sustainable core is being aware that there is a subtle layer of energy in the body. Yoga offers a map of how this energy might circulate. The mindful and energetic core practices are ones of cultivating awareness of this subtle energy layer. With an experienced teacher, we can learn to redirect our *prana* and optimize our health. We aim for our *agni*, or eternal flame, to burn steadily, but not flicker weakly nor rage out of control. Recall that there are many reasons why yoga "works," including the 5-fold (*panchamaya kosha*) and 3-fold (*gunas* and *polyvagal*) theories.[72] When we practice the 8 limbs of yoga, we have the opportunity to contemplate new ways of thinking with the moral lenses of the *yamas* and *niyamas*. I invite you and clients to consider practicing *ahimsa*, or non-violence, toward your body as you move through daily life, on and off the mat. I remind yoga students that we only get one body: treat it like a temple. Which means, we usually have a choice to practice non-violence to our body and non-self-harm which can reduce suffering. Being humble to the mysteries and making responsible choices and reactions to our situation are the final and most important element in activating your sustainable core. This is the secret sauce, the magic ingredient that will lead to integral health and well-being.

To simplify, I request every client to move mindfully with their breath. If they have discomfort with a given task, we break down the task into its physical components and explore pain-free ranges of motion. If we can't find comfortable movement, we start with centering the spine, modifying the load, and focus on reintegrating movements with the breath. Being stewards of our Earth-suits and cultivating a sustainable core is a lifetime practice. The more we consciously practice the individual parts in a quiet, safe space, the easier it might be to respond with resilience in stressful activities.

Part III

PRACTICES

9

IMPLEMENTING CHANGE VIA THERAPEUTIC EXERCISE

Let's put everything we have discussed together. While there are many layers and lenses to consider on the path to better health, one entry point is through our core layers. When we cultivate a sustainable core, we establish resilience and self-regulation through mindful breathing and movement. This is just one physical way into the center. This part provides instructions for individual practices that ultimately might be explored together, particularly mindful movement with breathing. When putting together an exercise and health plan, there are a few concepts to consider. I am not alone in finding success in using yoga as a tool to help people (including myself) feel better in their bodies.

Yoga and Healthy Lifestyles

It has long been known in yoga that living a healthy life includes eating and sleeping well. Some of the latest recommendations for mitigating chronic back pain include "lifestyle medicine strategies, such as incorporating whole foods and a plant-based diet, sustainable physical activity and mind-body exercises, restorative sleep, stress resiliency, awareness and mitigation of substance abuse and addiction, and establishing meaningful social networks and self-care strategies."[1] The benefits of yoga and the ingredients of healthy lifestyles are now being recommended by licensed health care providers, and the many layers of health are being recognized in the mainstream. The focus of this book is on the core, with the understanding that healthy changes are only achieved by simultaneously addressing the whole organism—including diet, sleep, spiritual wellness, and stress management.

The benefits of developing more control and coordination of the deep core muscles have recently entered the popular media, such as the article in the *New York Times* entitled "How simple exercises may save your lower back." The article notes that "Back pain is common and complicated. But altering your workout to build control and stability can help prevent it."[2] By now, I hope the lenses are clearer and the concepts seem within your grasp. When entering into a program to help ourselves and clients, in order to gradually build core control and stability, we should first consider where the client is, find a place of motor control, and then gradually and methodically introduce load, pacing, altered planes of gravity, and limb control.

Order of Exercise Progression
Graded Load and Pacing

As in cognitive behavioral therapy, pacing is a concept we use to build resilience and core stability. "Just as you wouldn't go outside and run a 26-mile-marathon tomorrow without training, you similarly wouldn't resume all physical activities after months at home with pain. 'Pacing' is a tried-and-true technique for slowly desensitizing brain and body, and gradually resuming your life."[3] So where does one begin? Start with a movement task and observe for compensations. If you have recovered from a back injury, have been cleared for exercise by your physician, and are ready to return to exercise.

I recommend gently practicing pain-free movement in the sagittal plane (flexion and extension) before introducing side-bending and rotation or twisting. "The position of the trunk has a significant impact on the ability to generate maximum intra-abdominal pressure during Valsalva's maneuver. Trunk rotation adversely affects this ability both in the flexed and standing positions."[4]

The body will often recruit helper muscles (and I propose that these muscles are the accessory breathing muscles) when the load or weight of a task is too much for our sustainable core to control our trunk. If we note that the accessory muscles are being recruited regularly in the gym, during activities of daily living, or on the mat, I suggest decreasing the load and retrying the task. Explore if the movement can be achieved without breath holding and without excessive accessory breathing muscle recruitment. Try finding a load and pace that reinforces dynamic stability from the sustainable core muscles. Once this control is found, this test turns into the homework or practice. Practice the task, mindfully, while breathing, and pace the movement with the sustainable core muscles moving in their homeostatic center without emergency core muscle recruitment.

Planes of Gravity and Developmental Progress

Another way to cultivate resilience and alter the load is by changing the body's position against gravity. Is the trunk stable with limb movement in all three planes of gravity? In other words, can the body perform movements without breath holding and emergency core muscle recruitment in supine exercises as well as prone and standing exercises?

What about moving through all the basic developmental patterns? Have you ever watched a baby learn to crawl and walk? There is a typical order of development we go through, from lying on our tummy, lifting and turning our head, engaging our wings, bending our hips and knees to crawl, crossing our limbs over the midline, kneeling, pulling to standing, cruising around the furniture, and, finally, walking. Ask yourself: are you capable of lying on the floor on your tummy, lifting your head, engaging your wings, crawling, kneeling, pulling to stand (lunge), and walking without your emergency breathing muscles being used for stability? If not, maybe start with some of the gentle exercises in this chapter first. Try static exercises (neutral spinal posture with no segmental displacement) before dynamic exercises (controlled spinal segmental movement).[5]

This is a gentle entry point for exploration. I don't intend to scare people into thinking that we should never use breath holding or our accessory breathing muscles as a strategy when faced with high loads. In fact, there is no evidence to suggest that high loads in exercise such as cross-fit lead to pelvic organ prolapse,[6, 7, 8] and physical therapists are reevaluating the premise that we should avoid high loads.[9] I am not saying we should avoid high loads; we just need to adjust, adapt, and use progressive, *gradual* progression of resistance. We have to meet the body where it is and figure out where it is compensating. In regard to activities with high loads, like cross-fit, physical therapist Julie Wiebe agrees: "Adaptive weight training strategies have their place to help build resilience as a way forward."[10] We just have to meet the body at its current level of ability and intervene, or work to change the strategy. This takes reorganization of thoughts and movement patterns, which takes time and mindfulness. I think the "secret sauce" to implementing this change is practicing mindful movement coordinated with breathing. I recommend learning novel breathing techniques, then applying them to, and coordinating them with, movement. I ask clients to check their center, sustainable core muscle coordination, breath, and awareness in every exercise and movement in daily life.

10

BREATHING EXERCISES

In learning breathing exercises, I recommend finding a quiet space without distractions where you can focus on what is going on in your internal environment. If you find aromatherapy beneficial, you might consider using a favorite scent you find relaxing or calming. It is safe to breathe in any position (remember, we are always using the diaphragm to breathe, so "abdominal breathing" is a bit of a misnomer). In all breathing exercises, we can alter the duration of any of the four parts of the breath cycle (the inhalation, pause, exhalation, and pause). As we learned in Chapter 6, The Breathing Core, expanding the length of the exhalation has many health benefits, including engaging the vagus nerve and increasing HRV. We start with an *even* inhalation and exhalation length, called a *box breath*.

BOX BREATH

- Sit or lie down in a comfortable position with your attention focused inwardly and breathe in and out through your nose.
- Begin counting after your next complete exhalation.
- Inhale for **two** counts.
- Pause at the top of the inhale for **two** counts.
- Exhale for **two** counts.
- Pause at the bottom of the exhale for **two** counts.
- Repeat for 3–10 cycles.
- Once this is accomplished with ease, try lengthening each

breath part to three seconds (that is, inhale for three seconds, pause for three seconds, exhale for three seconds, and pause for three seconds), then try four seconds each phase, and so on.

Lengthening the Exhalation

Once you feel comfortable with the box breath for four counts, try stretching out the exhalation for five or six counts and keep the rest of the counts the same.

- Sit or lie down in a comfortable position with your attention focused inwardly and breathe in and out through your nose.
- Begin counting the time after your next complete exhalation.
- Inhale for **four** counts.
- Pause at the top of the inhale for **four** counts.
- Exhale for **five to six** counts.
- Pause at the bottom of the exhale for **four** counts.
- Repeat for 3–10 cycles.

Once you are comfortable with that, try expanding the exhalation to seven counts, then eight counts, perhaps all the way up to nine or ten counts over several weeks or months or years of consistent practice. There is no rush, and as little as a few minutes per day can make a big shift in how one feels. Note how controlling the exhalation requires nuanced core muscle coordination.

You can also explore shortening or expanding the pause in between the inhale/exhale and vice versa. Keep your breathing even and smooth. If the 2–4 count feels too short, try increasing the breath lengths to **four** in and **six** out, **six** in and **eight** out, and so on. If longer breaths create any discomfort or agitation, there is no need to push yourself. The most important thing is that the exhale is longer than the inhale.

ALTERNATE NOSTRIL BREATHING (NADI SHODHANA)

As we have seen, breathing through the nose is healthier than mouth breathing. The most researched *pranayama* practice is alternate nostril breathing, or *nadi shodhana*. In Sanskrit, *"nadi"* = "channel," and *"shodhana"* = "cleaning or purifying." Simply put, it refers to the cleansing of the various channels in the human body using the technique of breath awareness. There are two variations of alternate nostril breathing: *anulom vilom*, where one consciously inhales through one nostril and exhales through the other, and *nadi shodhana*, where on the inhale, one holds the breaths for a brief period of time.[1]

Instructions

- Sit up tall and straight.
- Exhale completely through both nostrils and then use your right thumb to close your right nostril.
- Inhale through your left nostril, then pause while you close your left nostril with your right middle finger and open your right nostril by releasing your thumb.
- Exhale through your right nostril.
- Pause and keep your fingers and thumb in the same place.
- Inhale through your right nostril and then close this nostril with your thumb.
- Open your left nostril by releasing your finger and exhale through the left nostril.
- This is one cycle.
- Repeat the cycle for up to five minutes.
- It is traditional to complete the practice by finishing with an exhale through your left nostril, and then continue naturally breathing for several spontaneous cycles in and out of both nostrils.

ABDOMINO-DIAPHRAGMATIC BREATHING (BELLY BREATH)

Recall that the pelvic floor muscles, transverse abdominis muscle, and respiratory diaphragm muscles "wink," or pre-contract, with the thought of limb movement. For this reason, we want the limbs to remain relaxed during abdomino-diaphragmatic breathing in order to encourage relaxation and expansion, and allow increased length and range of motion in the PFM, TVA, and RD muscles.

Instructions

I recommend practicing this *pranayama* exercise in whatever position your body likes to take to encourage the abdominal muscles to relax. It is traditionally taught in a supine, or face-up, position. Some people prefer to do this in a modified child's pose, or face down with the forehead on the back of their hands. If you prefer to be on your back, try it with some pillows or towel rolls under your knees, lumbar spine, and neck as desired. Before you settle down, set a timer for 3–10 minutes (so you don't have to worry if you get too relaxed and fall asleep).

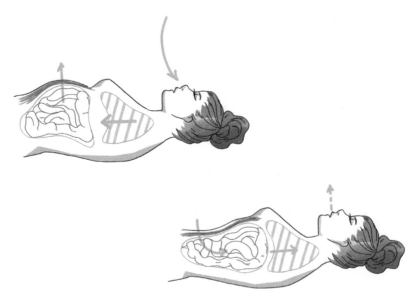

FIGURE 10.1 BELLY BREATH

- Find a comfortable, supported position, where you feel safe to relax your abdomen.
- If it's accessible in your chosen position, place one hand on your belly and the other on your chest or sternum.
- Use your hands to observe, without judgment, the movement or stillness of the abdomen and thorax.
- Imagine that all your muscles are melting into the floor as you breathe in and out (through your nose if possible).
- Do your best to maintain soft chest, neck, and facial muscles.
- At first, observe the location of the breath in the body. Do not try to change anything, just yet. Notice that you are breathing. Perhaps give a moment of gratitude to your Earth-suit for breathing for you all day long. You might say to yourself inwardly, "Way to go, body!"
- Now, bring your awareness to your abdomen rising toward the ceiling with the inhalation and passively (without muscular effort) lowering toward the ground with the exhalation. Do this for several more breath cycles.
- Begin to notice the pause between the inhale and exhale. Explore lingering in the stillness a moment before you exhale.
- Now, perhaps slow down the length of the exhalation.
- Note the stillness (or lack of it) at the end of the exhalation before you inhale again.
- With intention, deepen the expansion of the inhalation into the belly and explore keeping the movement in the chest to a minimum.

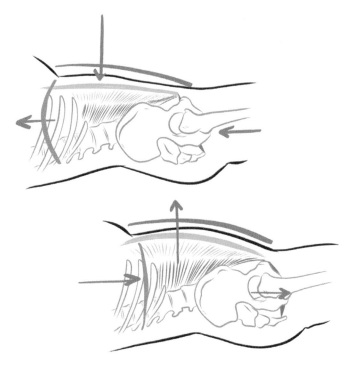

FIGURE 10.2 SUPINE BELLY BREATH

Options for Exploring "Belly Breath"

- Try pausing longer after a complete exhalation, before inhaling.
- Try pausing longer after fully inhaling, and allow the abdomen to naturally expand before exhaling.
- After ten conscious breath cycles, let go of the focus and simply rest the mind and body until the timer reminds you to return.
- If you like using rhythm and counting, explore using a metronome and count how many beats on your inhale, exhale, and pauses.
- Trauma-informed practitioners, or those who experience anxiety, report that using a weighted blanket or sandbag on their belly can be calming.
- Simply focus on allowing the respiratory diaphragm to expand to its full potential without taxing or stressing the chest muscles.

THORACO-DIAPHRAGMATIC BREATHING

Other names for this breath include band breath, wide breath, umbrella breath, jellyfish breath, mushroom breath, 360° breath, transversus abdominis-assisted thoraco-diaphragmatic breath, Pilates breath, and others. Remember that it is a respiratory diaphragm muscle breath (they all are!), with the emphasis on reversing the typical direction of the moving part (origin and insertion) of the respiratory diaphragm muscle. This requires some light muscle activation elsewhere in the sustainable core, typically the glottis or transverse abdominis. I typically prescribe it as a "stretch" or awareness exercise for improving the available range of motion of the RDM. It can be practiced in any position against gravity; I initially suggest a comfortable position other than lying on your back (because we want to allow full, available, excursion of the posterior ribs and RDM).

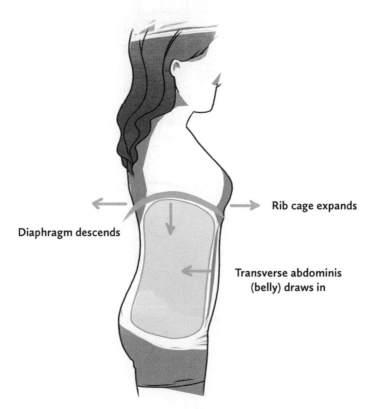

Rib cage expands

Diaphragm descends

Transverse abdominis (belly) draws in

FIGURE 10.3 THORACO-DIAPHRAGMATIC BREATH

Instructions

- Find a comfortable seated or prone position, where the lower ribs are free to expand posteriorly (behind you). Ideally, you would be in an alignment where the rib cage and pelvis line up (Figure 10.4).

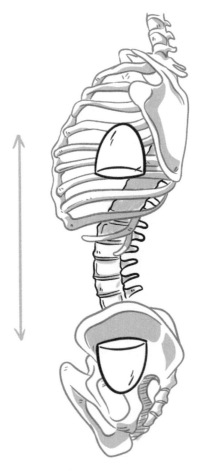

FIGURE 10.4 CLOSED EGG

- If seated or standing, lift your heart and crown toward the ceiling (axial extension) while grounding your sit bones or feet toward the earth.

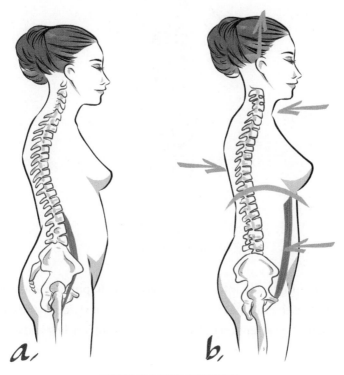

FIGURE 10.5 AXIAL EXTENSION

- If using a resistance band for tactile input, wrap it around the base of your ribs so it crosses in front, and tie it in a knot. Use your hands to feel the actual excursion of the lateral ribs (as shown). If your wrists are not comfortable in that position, don't tie the band, but cross it in front and hold the long sides of the band with your wrists straight and palms up (not shown).

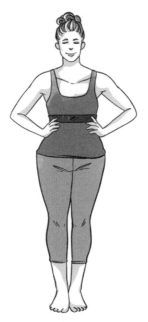

FIGURE 10.6 BAND BREATH

- Tune inwardly into your respiratory diaphragm muscle and notice the RD moving and breathing against your hands and/or band. Pay attention to the location of your inhaling and exhaling.

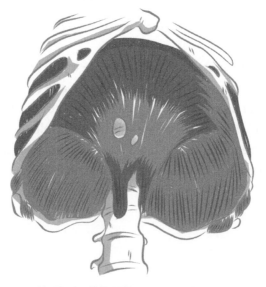

FIGURE 10.7 THE RESPIRATORY DIAPHRAGM

- On an inhalation, purposefully lengthen your entire spine. Maintain that length during the following breaths.
- Introduce a light TVA or glottal engagement (usually easier on the exhalation at first). Maintain the connection to the inner core muscles and consciously shift the expansion of the trunk from the belly to your back during the inhalation. Or simply continue to inhale while expanding the range of motion of your back and sides.
- Continue to attempt to "inhale into your back and sides" and expand the rib cage in all lateral dimensions. Do your best to avoid vertical motion, or elevation, of the collar bones and ribs.
- Imagine that your RD is an umbrella or jellyfish. Visualize the base of the umbrella or fish opening fully, in all 360 degrees of its diameter, with an *inhalation*.

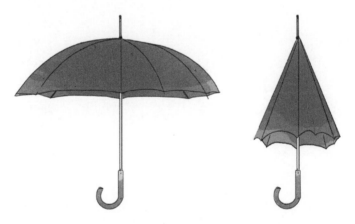

FIGURE 10.8 UMBRELLA

- The umbrella, jellyfish, or mushroom cap passively and easily closes the diameter of its base as you *exhale* with little to no effort.
- Continue to focus on the expansion of the diaphragm during the inhalation (this is where the intention can be placed).
- Continue inhaling into your lower ribs (wide and deep) and stay connected to your core during the inhalation *and* the exhalation phases of movement.

- Repeat for a few breaths.
- At first, I recommend 3–6 breaths, then work up to 6–10 in a session. Eventually, the goal is to be so proficient at this breath that you can consciously switch to it any time you need a little extra effort in life, at the gym, or on the mat. Or simply, any time you want to center your body, mind, and soul.

THREE-PART BREATH (*DIRGA PRANAYAMA*)

- Find a position where you can comfortably relax your abdomen. Ideally, recline on a soft surface to allow room for the posterior ribs to expand as well as the belly.
- Place one hand on your heart/sternum and the other on your belly.
- Take a deep breath, filling the bony core cylinder from the base to the top.
- In sequence:
  - Slowly inhale through your nose and observe the breath coming in through the nasal tube and down through the lungs, into your belly and pelvis (part one).
  - When the abdomen and pelvis are expanded, direct the inhalation into the sides and back of the ribs (part two).
  - Then, allow the sternum, chest, upper ribs, and lower throat to fill and stretch (part three).
- Stop inhaling before you feel any strain; a gentle stretching sensation is optimal.
- Pause consciously at the top of the inhalation.
- Exhale passively, allowing all three chambers to empty together.
- Pause consciously at the bottom of the exhale.
- Repeat with the aim of lengthening and deepening the inhalation.
- At first, you will want to focus on isolating the movement in and out of the three sections, monitoring the movement with your hands.
- Over time, you might have a better internal feel for the breath and not want to use the hands.
- Work toward continuously breathing in and out of the three chambers as one unit from the bottom up, like a wave.
- Another way to think about this is to imagine that your bony core canister has rings on its sides stacked all the way from the bottom to the top of the can. Visualize expanding the diameter of those rings, one at a time, from the bottom to the top. You

can imagine three rings, and over time, work on increasing the number of rings up to as many as you have time for.

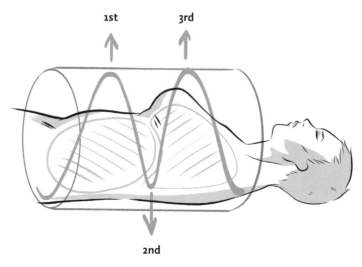

FIGURE 10.9 *DIRGA PRANAYAMA*

UJJAYI BREATH (CONTROLLED GLOTTAL BREATH)

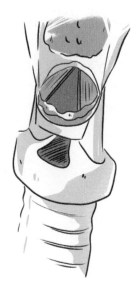 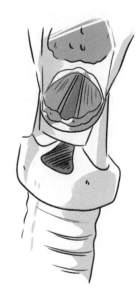

FIGURE 10.10 THE GLOTTIS

- Begin in any comfortable position.
- For best airway access, initially align the head so it is centered on the thorax (recall the snow-person posture) or avoid excessive forward head posture.
- Turn your attention inwardly and focus on your throat.
- Notice the breath passing in and out of the throat and through the vocal folds.
- On an *exhalation*, lightly close the base of the throat to create a "*ha*" sound.
- Continue to breathe in and out softly and slowly and explore this "*ha*" sound with the exhalation, as if you were fogging up a mirror. Can you maintain the sound throughout the entire exhalation? Does it sound like water rushing or an ocean wave?
- At first, it is usually easier to modulate the volume and intensity of the sound with the mouth open. Can you also subtly make that sound with your mouth closed?

- Once you master the control of the sound with the exhalation and the mouth closed, try creating the same sound during the *inhalation*.
- Explore making a soft sound with your mouth closed on the inhalation *and* the exhalation.
- Once you accomplish this breath at rest, try applying it to tasks that require effort (like lifting, pushing, or pulling) or during transitions between poses/*asanas* on the mat.

11

THERAPEUTIC PHYSICAL–
ENERGETIC PRACTICES

REVERSE KEGEL (PFM AWARENESS)

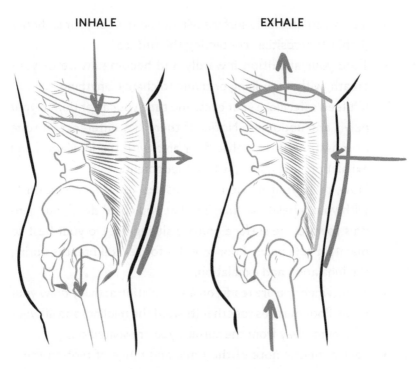

INHALE

EXHALE

FIGURE 11.1 STANDING REVERSE KEGEL

This exercise can be performed in any position. If the intention is to relax, then I recommend practicing it lying down. If the goal is for awareness, you might receive more tactile input by practicing this in a seated position—perhaps even sitting on a folded towel or washcloth under your perineum for increased tactile input.

No matter what position you choose, make yourself comfortable and do what feels best in this moment.

In any supported position, tune inward and observe your breath. Consciously relax and allow the pelvic floor muscles to soften and "drop" on an inhalation. Exhale while remaining relaxed in the pelvic floor and abdominals (the muscles should subtly recoil back to the starting length without effort; don't panic if nothing seems to happen automatically—we are observing without judgment). Repeat, continuing to relax the PFM on the inhalation, 3–6 times in a session.

How to self-assess pelvic floor muscle recruitment and length:

- Sit on a comfortable surface with awareness of your sit bones (ischial tuberosities) contacting the surface.
- Tune your attention inwardly and become aware of your breath, without judging or trying to change anything.
- If it feels safe, close your eyes, and tune your attention to your pelvis and abdomen. Notice if there is a difference in tone or sensation of the pelvic floor area with the inhalation and exhalation. Just notice, without judgment.
- Now, relax your pelvic floor muscles and TVA consciously with your inhalation. Imagine that you could drop your genitals toward the surface you are sitting on. Do your best to maintain soft pelvic floor muscles for several breaths during the inhalation and exhalation.
- Then, when you are ready, on an exhalation actively draw your pelvic floor muscles together (toward the midline) and lift your perineum away from the surface you are seated on.
- Take a mental note of the force and range of motion these muscles are capable of.
- Relax the muscles again.
- Place your hands on your lower abdomen and "listen" with your hands for movement or stillness.

- With your hands on your abdomen, try contracting the PFM again on your exhalation. When you contract your pelvic floor muscles, do the abdominal muscles respond?
- If there is no pain or discomfort, try coordinating the contraction and relaxation with the breath.

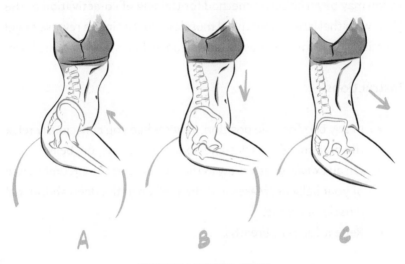

FIGURE 11.2 NEUTRAL PELVIS

Now, try the above PFM contraction and relaxation in a posteriorly tucked position of the pelvis (position C). Then, try again in an anteriorly tilted pelvis position (position A). Reflect: Which position allowed for the greatest force generation and range of motion of the muscles for you today? Generally, the PFM have the best length-tension relationship in neutral.

TRANSVERSE ABDOMINIS RECRUITMENT WITH BELLY BREATH

Next, try relaxing the transverse abdominis muscle (TVA) followed by a deliberate contraction of the TVA with a strong exhalation. Ishida, Hirose, and Watanabe conclude in their study that "Maximum expiration may be an effective method for training of co-activation of the [TVA with the] lateral abdominal muscles."[1] Just as in the reverse Kegel exercise, this isometric muscle activation includes a relaxation phase.

Instructions

- In any comfortable position, *inhale* while you consciously relax the abdominal muscles and abdominal tissue, or "belly."
- On an *exhale*, gently draw in the TVA so that the circumference of your belly decreases and the tension in the deep abdominal muscles increase.
- Repeat for 3–10 breaths.

Note that sometimes people ask what the difference is between this and a reverse Kegel. The answer is almost nothing, except for which muscles are relaxing and engaging. A reverse Kegel is the relaxation and contraction of the *pelvic floor muscles* in sync with the breath. A TVA brace is a relaxation and contraction of the *transverse abdominis muscle* in sync with the breath. If you have accomplished the controlled reverse Kegel exercise and the TVA engagement exercises successfully separately, now try them together: relax both the PFM and TVA on the inhalation and lightly contract them both with the exhalation.

TVA VERSUS RECTUS ABDOMINIS RECRUITMENT

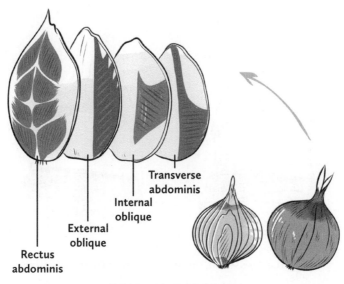

FIGURE 11.3 THE TVA ONION

When learning how to control the deep transverse abdominis muscle, sometimes the superficial rectus abdominis muscle responds first. One of the main aims of this book is to include the deep TVA as the first responder in the sustainable core muscle team. Place your fingers just to the side of the rectus abdominis muscle: Is there any tension deep in the TVA? Or is that space soft and mushy? Work with the full exhalation to recruit the deep TVA. Feel into the movement. Check to see that your deep abdominal muscles are drawing in and flattening like the muscles on the left in Figure 11.4. Watch for the rectus abdominis muscle doming (and try to avoid the doming or gathering that you see on the right in Figure 11.4).

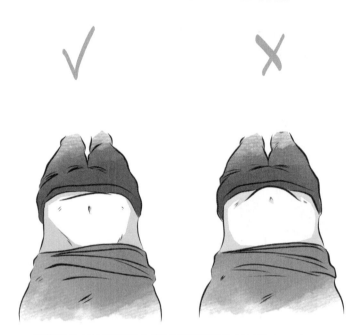

FIGURE 11.4 TRANSVERSE ABDOMINIS VERSUS RECTUS ABDOMINIS

SCAPULAR RETRACTION AND DEPRESSION IN NEUTRAL SPINE

For regaining control of the upper core, simply isolating the scapula or moving the arms, while maintaining neutral spine, can be challenging. Once accomplished, deep rewards are often discovered. (Spoiler Alert: control of the deep, superior transverse abdominis muscle fibers helps with this task.)

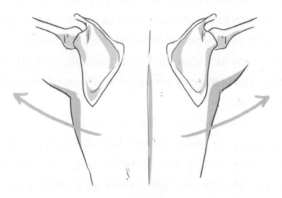

FIGURE II.5 UPWARD ROTATION OF THE SCAPULA

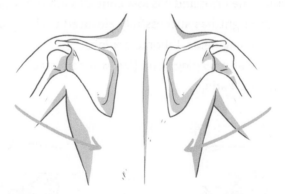

FIGURE II.6 DOWNWARD ROTATION OF THE SCAPULA

Instructions

- Either lie on your back on a foam roller (with the roller parallel to the spine) and your knees bent, or stand with a foam roller placed vertically between your spine and the wall. This position is similar to the position of the broomstick or dowel in the discussion of posture in Chapter 4, The Bony Core. Note that the same three points would be in contact with the roller as the dowel: the head, the mid-thoracic spine (T8 or so), and the mid-sacrum.

- Elevate your arms so your hands rise above your head (shoulder flexion).
- Pause and stop elevating your arms *before* you note any pinching or radiating pain.
- If your shoulders have full, pain-free range of motion, can you flex your shoulders to 180° without losing neutral spine? Can you maintain neutral pelvis? What happens if you engage your wings?
- Explore what happens if you maintain neutral spine on the foam roller, engage your upper and lower TVA, and move with your breath.
- If you are on a foam roller, are you able to maintain contact between your midback and the roller (approximately where a bra strap, or thoracic vertebra, might be)? In other words, can you elevate your arms without arching your midback or flaring your ribs? See Figure 11.7, where the figure on the left is flaring their ribs and has lost contact with the wall. The figure on the right has successfully elevated their shoulders while maintaining neutral thoracic spine.
- Note that engaging your TVA will help stabilize the ribs and minimize flaring.

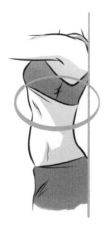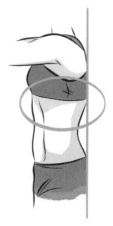

FIGURE 11.7 RIB FLARE

SUPINE MARCHING

This exercise is part of a classic core progression series,[2] and can also be called "hook-lying (on your back, knees bent) static (isometric or not moving) TVA march."

Instructions

- Lie on your back on the floor in neutral spine with your knees bent and your feet on the floor.
- Use your thumbs to monitor your lower ribs, your pinky fingers to monitor your anterior pelvis points (ASIS), and your middle fingers to feel your abdominal muscle.
- Take a preparatory *inhalation* into your side ribs without moving your spine.
- On the *exhale*, in sequence: engage your deep core muscles (PFM, TVA, and "wings"), and then lift one knee toward your chest in coordination with the exhalation.
- Monitor your neutral pelvis and abdominal control with your fingers.
- Pause and breathe in and out with one knee in the air until you are steady.
- Maintain trunk stability and a steady breath during the transition to the other leg.
- Repeat on the other leg.

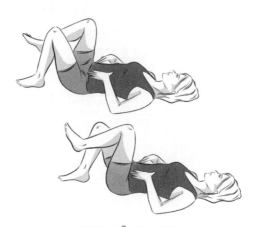

FIGURE 11.8 TVA MARCH

- Pretend that you have a teacup with hot tea balanced on your belly. Can you control the imaginary teacup on your stable belly with your core while breathing into your back and sides?
- If this is too easy for you, try it while lying on a foam roller (with your spine parallel to the roll). Can you lift one leg off the floor and breathe steadily without falling off the roller? Check: Are you breathing into your thorax? (That is, are you using a thoraco-diaphragmatic breath?) Are you able to maintain relaxation of the accessory breathing muscles?
- If you can maintain a steady breath on the foam roller without substituting IAP or accessory breathing muscles for compensation, then try "marching" in coordination with your breath. *Exhale as you lift one leg, pause, and inhale while you lower that leg to the floor.* Then, exhale while you bring the other knee toward the chest and inhale to lower that leg. Continue "marching" in coordination with your breath for 10–20 "steps."
- The creative progressions are countless. To increase the load, we could extend an arm overhead and/or straighten the opposite knee towards a classic "dead bug" rehabilitation exercise. Increasing the lever arm increases the demand of the core muscles and we can increase or decrease the lever arm to meet the needs of the body we are working with.

NEUTRAL SPINE POSTURE IN QUADRUPED

I recommend this assessment for people who want to return to fitness or yoga classes that involve planks or push-ups. Can you find a neutral spine shape comfortably on your hands and knees?

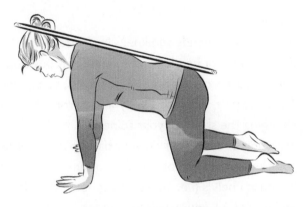

FIGURE 11.9 QUADRUPED WITH DOWEL

Try using a dowel, broomstick, or foam roller parallel to the spine to check the curves. Kneel on a soft surface to protect your knees. If the wrists don't have enough range or strength for this position, try weight-bearing on your elbows and forearms instead (see Figure 11.10). Pause and breathe here for 6–10 thoraco-diaphragmatic breaths. Can you find the spinal shape without relying on the dowel?

PREGNANT CAT

Otherwise known as "transverse abdominis muscle brace and relaxation in quadruped," or simply "belly breathing plus TVA contraction in quadruped."

Instructions

- Begin on your hands and knees in neutral spine.
- If your wrists or hands don't tolerate this position, try placing your forearms on the floor or on blocks, as shown.
- On an *exhale*, draw the belly away from the floor without changing the shape of your spine.
- Try using a foam roller on your back, placed perpendicular to your lumbar spine (not shown), to remind yourself to remain in neutral pelvis (i.e., don't let the roller fall off of your back, and don't tuck your pelvis/tail under).
- On an *inhale*, relax your belly without changing the shape of your spine.
- *Exhale* and draw the belly in again. Repeat 3–10 times.

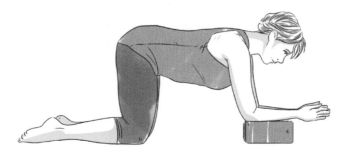

FIGURE II.IO QUADRUPED ON FOREARMS

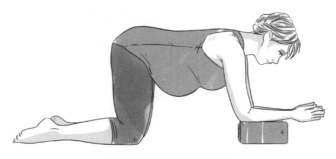

FIGURE II.II PREGNANT CAT

Now, can you maintain this neutral shape of the spine and perform a *thoraco-diaphragmatic breath* in this position? Next, try it with a dowel parallel to the spine. Can you maintain thoracic contact with the dowel throughout an entire breath cycle? (That is, do you lose contact with the dowel at your midback during the inhalation or exhalation?) Note that the TVA will slightly lengthen during the inhalation and contract during the exhalation. Can you maintain a midrange TVA muscle contraction with this slight fluctuation with the breath without totally letting go of the abdominal muscles, or without a 100 percent/maximal contraction as well?

Once you can breathe smoothly while maintaining neutral spine in this quadruped position, try a little movement. Can you maintain contact with the dowel while lifting one hand off the floor? And, are you able to continue breathing smoothly throughout the movement?

What happens if you switch hands?

Can you extend one leg behind you and the opposite arm out in front of you (while breathing and maintaining contact with the dowel)?

Test your control while switching to the opposite arm and leg. Can you maintain neutral spine while breathing during the transition? The variations are numerous, but this task should start to look like the traditional "bird dog" spinal stabilization exercise in typical rehabilitation settings, but without breath-holding or deviating from a neutral spine shape.

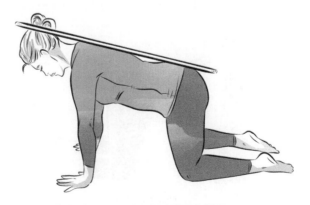

FIGURE 11.12 QUADRUPED WITH DOWEL

QUADRUPED SPINAL EXTENSION AND FLEXION (CAT AND COW)

Note that this exercise is not in neutral spine.

Instructions

- Begin on your hands and knees, with your hands under your shoulders and a blanket under your knees.
- Lightly engage your "wings" by activating the muscles at the lower part of your scapulae. Externally rotate your humerus so that your elbow crease is moving toward the front of the mat and away from your midline. Maintain soft (not locked) elbows throughout the spinal movements.
- *Inhale* as you extend your spine (head, heart, and tail up as the back arches down). Slide your shoulder blades together and down your back (scapular *depression + retraction*).
- Try not to hinge or fold the skin in your neck. Instead, keep the neck long (axial extension) and explore gazing between your hands or toward the top of the mat rather than at the wall in front of you.
- *Exhale* as you flex your spine, tuck your pelvis, and draw your abdominals in (head and tail tuck down as your spine arches up). Broaden your shoulder blades and push your hands into the mat to hollow out your armpits (scapular *protraction*).

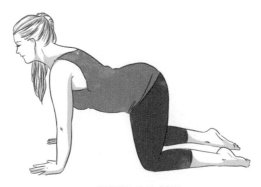

FIGURE II.I3 COW

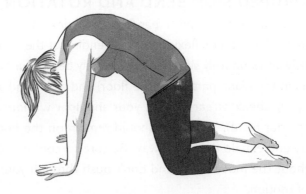

FIGURE 11.14 CAT

Repeat with your breath (inhaling with extension/cow and exhaling with flexion/cat) 6–10 times. Once you accomplish this, try reversing the breath (inhale during cat and exhale during cow). Note how switching up the breath affects the subtle energy flow.

QUADRUPED SIDE-BEND AND ROTATION

Explore: Once you accomplish fear-free spinal flexion and extension (cat and cow), try lateral flexion or side-bending of the spine.

Gently and smoothly side-bend or laterally bend your pelvis (wag your tail in the plane parallel to the floor) and side-bend your neck (move your cheek or ear toward your shoulder without turning/rotating your head). Your gaze should remain on the floor. Inhale one way and exhale the other way. Be sure to continue breathing throughout the movements and don't push through your comfort range of motion.

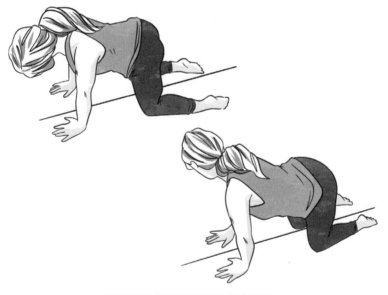

FIGURE II.I5 QUADRUPED SIDE-BEND

Now that you have moved through flexion, extension, and side-bending of the spine in quadruped, explore rotation of the spine. Try raising your hand to the side (technically termed "shoulder horizontal abduction"), while rotating your thorax or twisting your trunk, so that your hand or elbow and shoulder blade move toward the ceiling. Follow your hand with your eyes and head and look up toward the ceiling to a gentle stretch point. Pause and breathe steadily. Place your hand back on the floor in neutral spine and repeat on the other side. Once you are comfortable pausing and breathing in the twist, practice moving mindfully with your breath while rotating and switching hands, a few times each way.

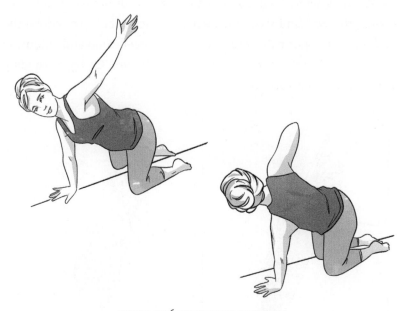

FIGURE 11.16 QUADRUPED ROTATION

STANDING THORAX ROTATION AT THE WALL

If your body does not tolerate weight-bearing on its hands and knees, you can experience the same spinal positions and breaths in standing. Try standing while facing a wall and place your hands or forearms against the wall and step your feet 6–12 inches back to reduce the load on your upper-extremities. Explore spinal flexion and extension (cat and cow) with your knees bent (not shown). Or try a standing plank on wall plus rotation.

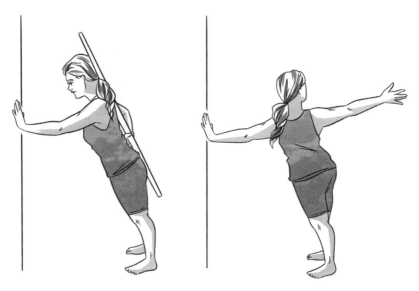

FIGURE 11.17 WALL PLANK PLUS THORAX ROTATION
PLANK ON FOREARMS

If you can tolerate all the above exercises without exacerbating symptoms, while breathing, another way to increase the load or weight on the core is by increasing the lever arm against gravity, as in traditional planks.

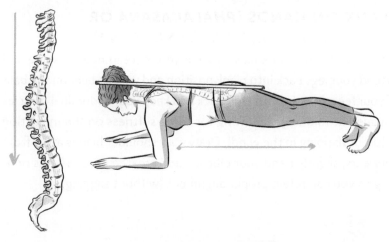

FIGURE 11.18 PLANK ON ELBOWS

PLANK ON HANDS (*PHALAKASANA* OR *UTTIHITA CHATURANGA DANDASANA*)

From your hands and knees, engage your core in neutral spine and extend your legs back into plank position and weight-bear on the balls of your feet. Breathe into your back and keep your abdominal muscles engaged at midrange, allowing for some softness on the inhalation (without flapping in the wind). Draw your shoulder blades away from your ears, slightly bend your elbows, and breathe 6–10 breaths or as long as you can retain proper alignment (without sagging).

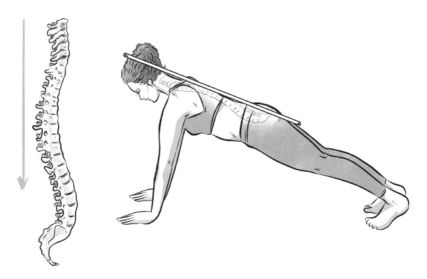

FIGURE 11.19 PLANK ON HANDS

DOWNWARD-FACING DOG (*ADHO MUKHA SVANASANA*)

From plank on hands, bend your knees, and lift your hips towards the ceiling (hip flexion) while pushing your hands into the floor and flexing your shoulders, shifting to downward-facing dog pose. Try energetically activating your arm muscles. Try spreading your fingers and maintain connection to your wings (keep the muscles engaged at midrange). Imagine pushing the floor down and forward. If you can maintain neutral spine, slowly lower your heels toward the ground or explore stepping your hands and feet closer together. Maintain spinal length and axial extension by lengthening your crown and tailbone in opposite directions. Pause and breathe for 6–10 breaths.

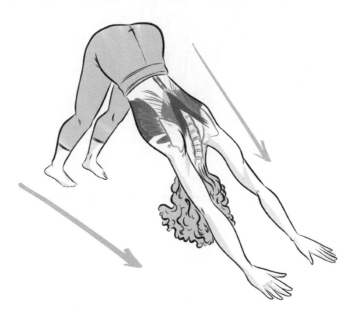

FIGURE 11.20 DOWNWARD-FACING DOG WINGS

MOUNTAIN POSE (*TADASANA*)

Can you stand with upright posture with your back against the wall or with a dowel honoring the neutral curves of the spine?

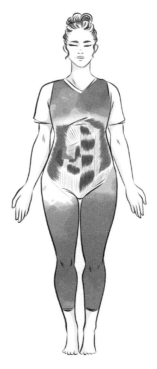

FIGURE 11.21 MOUNTAIN POSE (WITH THE ABDOMINALS SHOWN)

STANDING SIDE-BENDS

Try spinal side-bending with your hands on heart (in prayer *mudra*) and/or with your hands overhead.

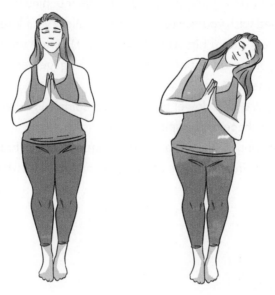

FIGURE 11.22 HANDS ON HEART

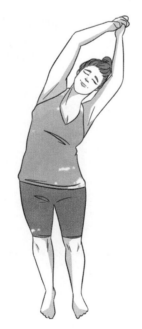

FIGURE 11.23 ARMS OVERHEAD

CHAIR POSE (A VARIATION OF *UTKATASANA*)

From mountain pose, engage your core and bend your ankles, knees, and hips to slightly shift your pelvis behind you and your torso forward, as if you were going to sit down in a chair behind you. Keep your knees aligned with your second toes (don't allow your knees to come together, keep them hip-width throughout). Bring your arms only as high as you can maintain scapular/wing engagement and neutral spine. Breathe for 6–10 breaths.

Now, try it with a dowel to check your spinal alignment. Can you maintain the shape of the spine while transitioning in and out of the pose? What about while you are in the posture, can you breathe in and out without losing the shape of the spine or contact with the dowel?

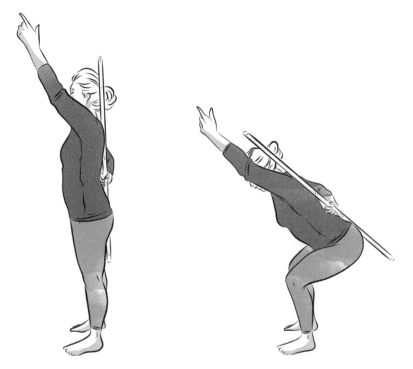

FIGURE II.24 CHAIR POSE WITH DOWEL

FUNCTIONAL SQUAT

Finally, putting it all together, can you maintain neutral spine and pick up a pencil or a heavy box from the floor while holding the dowel on the spine, without holding your breath?

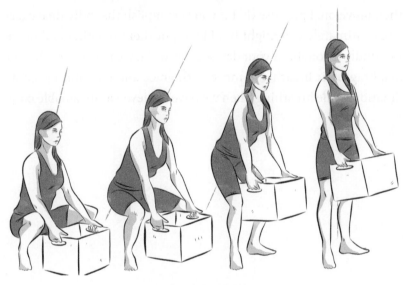

FIGURE 11.25 BOX SQUAT

If not, we may need to look at your limbs, investigate further, or seek guidance from a medical provider to help you regain your range of motion, strength, and functional mobility to live life with less suffering.

The exercises presented here are dissectible parts of a whole body in motion. When the individual pieces are running smoothly, the entire machine is more efficient. I present the exercises in a progressive format that allows you to safely find your strengths and weaknesses. When you find yourself challenged by an exercise, practice it a bit and then move on. I propose that if you accomplish the individual exercises, ultimately you might be able to put them together and move mindfully throughout your day. Ideally, when we master an efficient diaphragmatic breath and move with grace and core muscle coordination while breathing, then we have achieved a sustainable core.

References

Foreword

1   Nicholls, David A. (2017). *The End of Physiotherapy*. London: Routledge. p. 2.

Chapter 1

1   Kibler, W. B., Press, J., & Sciascia, A. (2006). The role of core stability in athletic function. *Sports Medicine, 36*(3), 189–198.

2   Saeterbakken, A. H., Stien, N., Pedersen, H., & Andersen, V. (2022). Core muscle activation in three lower extremity exercises with different stability requirements. *Journal of Strength and Conditioning Research, 36*(2), 304–309.

3   Zoffness, R. (2019). A tale of two nails. *Psychology Today*. Accessed on July 9, 2022 at www.psychologytoday.com/us/blog/pain-explained/201911/tale-two-nails.

4   Kilic, O., Maas, M., Verhagen, E., Zwerver, J., & Gouttebarge, V. (2017). Incidence, aetiology and prevention of musculoskeletal injuries in volleyball: A systematic review of the literature. *European Journal of Sport Science, 17*(6), 765–793.

5   Lawrence, R. C., Felson, D. T., Helmick, C. G., Arnold, L. M., et al. (2008). Estimates of the prevalence of arthritis and other rheumatic conditions in the United States: Part II. *Arthritis and Rheumatism, 58*(1), 26–35.

6   Nelson, A. E., Allen, K. D., Golightly, Y. M., Goode, A. P., & Jordan, J. M. (2014). A systematic review of recommendations and guidelines for the management of osteoarthritis: The chronic osteoarthritis management initiative of the US bone and joint initiative. *Seminars in Arthritis and Rheumatism, 43*(6), 701–712.

7   Sinnott, P. L., Dally, S. K., Trafton, J., Goulet, J. L., & Wagner, T. H. (2017). Trends in diagnosis of painful neck and back conditions, 2002 to 2011. *Medicine, 96*(20), e6691.

8   Pearson, N., Prosko, S., Sullivan, M., & Taylor, M. J. (2020). White Paper: Yoga therapy and pain—how yoga therapy serves in comprehensive integrative pain management, and how it can do more. *International Journal of Yoga Therapy, 30*(1), 117–133.

9   Frogner, B. K., Harwood, K., Andrilla, C. H. A., Schwartz, M., & Pines, J. M. (2018). Physical therapy as the first point of care to treat low back pain: An instrumental variables approach to estimate impact on opioid prescription, health care utilization, and costs. *Journal of Health Services Research and Policy, 53*(6), 4629–4646.

10 US Department of Health and Human Services (2019). *Pain Management Best Practices Inter-Agency Task Force Report: Updates, Gaps, Inconsistencies, and Recommendations*. New York: US Department of Health and Human Services. Accessed

on January 4, 2023 at www.hhs.gov/sites/default/files/pmtf-final-report-2019-05-23. pdf.

11 Wainner, R. S., Whitman, J. M., Cleland, J. A., & Flynn, T. W. (2007). Regional interdependence: A musculoskeletal examination model whose time has come. *Journal of Orthopaedic and Sports Physical Therapy*, *37*(11), 658–660.

12 Sueki, D. G., Cleland, J. A., & Wainner, R. S. (2013). A regional interdependence model of musculoskeletal dysfunction: Research, mechanisms, and clinical implications. *Journal of Manual and Manipulative Therapy*, *21*(2), 90–102.

13 Wims, M. E., McIntyre, S. M., York, A., & Covill, L. G. (2017). The use of yoga by physical therapists in the United States. *International Journal of Yoga Therapy*, *27*(1), 69–79. p. 69.

14 Defreese, J. D. (2017). Athlete mental health care within the biopsychosocial model. *Athletic Training and Sports Health Care*, *9*(6), 243–245.

15 Engel, G. L. (1980). The clinical application of the biopsychosocial model. *American Journal of Psychiatry*, *137*(5), 535–544.

16 Evans, S., Tsao, J. C., Sternlieb, B., & Zeltzer, L. K. (2009). Using the biopsychosocial model to understand the health benefits of yoga. *Journal of Complementary and Integrative Medicine*, *6*(1), 1–22.

17 Gatchel, R. J., Peng, Y. B., Peters, M. L., Fuchs, P. N., & Turk, D. C. (2007). The biopsychosocial approach to chronic pain: Scientific advances and future directions. *Psychological Bulletin*, *133*(4), 581–624.

18 Kersting, K. (2005). A chorus of voices for the biopsychosocial model. *Monitor on Psychology*, *36*(5). Accessed on March 14, 2018 at www.apa.org/monitor/may05/ voices.aspx.

19 Borell-Carrió, F., Suchman, A. L., & Epstein, R. M. (2004). The biopsychosocial model 25 years later: Principles, practice, and scientific inquiry. *Annals of Family Medicine*, *2*, 576–582.

20 Foster, N. E., & Delitto, A. (2011). Embedding psychosocial perspectives within clinical management of low back pain: Integration of psychosocially informed management principles into physical therapist practice—challenges and opportunities. *Physical Therapy*, *91*(5), 790–803.

21 Taylor, M. (2012). Creating a biopsychosocial bridge of care: Linking yoga therapy and medical rehabilitation. *International Journal of Yoga Therapy*, *22*, 93–94.

22 Pearson, N., Prosko, S., Sullivan, M., & Taylor, M. J. (2020). White Paper: Yoga therapy and pain—how yoga therapy serves in comprehensive integrative pain management, and how it can do more. *International Journal of Yoga Therapy*, *30*(1), 117–133.

23 Taylor, M., & Milson, H. (2017) Week 1 class outline: Introduction to yoga therapeutics. Session 1 of Integrating yoga therapeutics into rehabilitation [Online course].

24 Stilwell, P., & Harman, K. (2019). An enactive approach to pain: Beyond the biopsychosocial model. *Phenomenology and the Cognitive Sciences*, *18*(4), 637–665.

25 Mescouto, K., Olson, R. E., Hodges, P. W., & Setchell, J. (2022). A critical review of the biopsychosocial model of low back pain care: Time for a new approach? *Disability and Rehabilitation*, *44*(13), 3270–3284.

26 Stilwell, P., & Harman, K. (2019). An enactive approach to pain: Beyond the biopsychosocial model. *Phenomenology and the Cognitive Sciences*, *18*(4), 637–665.

27 Wims, M. E., McIntyre, S. M., York, A., & Covill, L. G. (2017). The use of yoga by physical therapists in the United States. *International Journal of Yoga Therapy*, *27*(1), 69–79.

28 Pearson, N., Prosko, S., Sullivan, M., & Taylor, M. J. (2020). White Paper: Yoga therapy and pain—how yoga therapy serves in comprehensive integrative pain

management, and how it can do more. *International Journal of Yoga Therapy, 30*(1), 117–133.

Chapter 2

1   Bhavanani, A. B., & Ramanathan, M. (2018). Psychophysiology of Yoga Postures: Ancient and Modern Perspectives of Asanas. In S. Telles & N. Singh (eds.) *Research-Based Perspectives on the Psychophysiology of Yoga* (pp. 1–16). Hershey, PA: IGI Global.

2   Jeter, P. E., Slutsky, J., Singh, N., & Khalsa, S. B. S. (2015). Yoga as a therapeutic intervention: A bibliometric analysis of published research studies from 1967 to 2013. *Journal of Alternative and Complementary Medicine, 21*(10), 586–592.

3   Brown, R. P., & Gerberg, P. L. (2005). Sudarshan Kriya yogic breathing in the treatment of stress, anxiety, and depression: Part I—neurophysiologic model. *Journal of Alternative and Complementary Medicine, 11*, 189–201.

4   Cabral, P., Meyer, H. B., & Ames, D. (2011). Effectiveness of yoga therapy as a complementary treatment for major psychiatric disorders: A meta-analysis. *The Primary Care Companion to CNS Disorders, 13*(4), PCC.10r01068.

5   Smith, C., Hancock, H., Blake-Mortimer, J., & Eckert, K. (2007). A randomised comparative trial of yoga and relaxation to reduce stress and anxiety. *Complementary Therapies in Medicine, 15*(2), 77–83.

6   Khalsa, S. B. (2007). Yoga as a therapeutic intervention. *Principles and Practice of Stress Management, 3*, 449–462.

7   Bower, J. E., Greendale, G., Crosswell, A. D., Garet, D., et al. (2014). Yoga reduces inflammatory signaling in fatigued breast cancer survivors: A randomized controlled trial. *Psychoneuroendocrinology, 43*, 20–29.

8   Field, T. (2016). Yoga research review. *Complementary Therapies in Clinical Practice, 24*, 145–161.

9   Field, T. (2016). Yoga research review. *Complementary Therapies in Clinical Practice, 24*, 145–161.

10 Field, T. (2016). Yoga research review. *Complementary Therapies in Clinical Practice, 24*, 145–161.

11 Field, T. (2016). Yoga research review. *Complementary Therapies in Clinical Practice, 24*, 145–161.

12 Cramer, H., Quinker, D., Schumann, D., Wardle, J., et al. (2019). Adverse effects of yoga: A national cross-sectional survey. *BioMed Central Complementary and Alternative Medicine, 19*(1), 1–10.

13 Field, T. (2016). Yoga research review. *Complementary Therapies in Clinical Practice, 24*, 145–161.

14 Bhavanani, A. B., & Ramanathan, M. (2018). Psychophysiology of Yoga Postures: Ancient and Modern Perspectives of Asanas. In S. Telles & N. Singh (eds.) *Research-Based Perspectives on the Psychophysiology of Yoga* (pp. 1–16). Hershey, PA: IGI Global. p. 1.

15 Bhavanani, A. B., & Ramanathan, M. (2018). Psychophysiology of Yoga Postures: Ancient and Modern Perspectives of Asanas. In S. Telles & N. Singh (eds.) *Research-Based Perspectives on the Psychophysiology of Yoga* (pp. 1–16). Hershey, PA: IGI Global.

16 Payne, L., Gold, T., & Goldman, E. (2015). *Yoga Therapy and Integrative Medicine: Where Ancient Science Meets Modern Medicine.* Laguna Beach, CA: Basic Health Publications. p. 28.

17 Carrico, M. (2021, March 23). Get to know the 8 limbs of yoga. *Yoga Journal*. Accessed on February 11, 2022 at www.yogajournal.com/yoga-101/philosophy/8-limbs-of-yoga/eight-limbs-of-yoga.

18 Satchidananda, S. (1984). *The Yoga Sutras of Patanjali: Translation and Commentary by Sri Swami Satchidananda*. Yogaville, VA: Integral Yoga Publications. Sutra 2.46. p. 152.

Chapter 3

1   Willardson, J. M. (2007). Core stability training: Applications to sports conditioning programs. *Journal of Strength and Conditioning Research*, *21*(3), 979–985.
2   Behm, D. G., Drinkwater, E. J., Willardson, J. M., & Cowley, P. M. (2010). The use of instability to train the core musculature. *Applied Physiology, Nutrition, and Metabolism*, *35*(1), 91–108.
3   Physical Solutions (2015). *Understanding Planes and Axes of Movement*. Ingoldisthorpe, Norfolk: Physical Solutions. Accessed on October 1, 2022 at www.physical-solutions.co.uk/wp-content/uploads/2015/05/Understanding-Planes-and-Axes-of-Movement.pdf.
4   Vlaeyen, J. W., Crombez, G., & Linton, S. J. (2016). The fear-avoidance model of pain. *Pain*, *157*(8), 1588–1589.

Chapter 4

1   Kapandji, A. I. (2019). *The Physiology of the Joints, Volume 3: The Spinal Column, Pelvic Girdle and Head*. Pencaitland, East Lothian: Handspring Publishing.
2   Panjabi, M. M. (1992). The stabilizing system of the spine. Part II. Neutral zone and instability hypothesis. *Journal of Spinal Disorders*, *5*, 390–396.
3   Sapsford, R. R., Richardson, C. A., Maher, C. F., & Hodges, P. W. (2008). Pelvic floor muscle activity in different sitting postures in continent and incontinent women. *Archives of Physical Medicine and Rehabilitation*, *89*(9), 1741–1747.
4   Claus, A. P., Hides, J. A., Moseley, G. L., & Hodges, P. W. (2009). Different ways to balance the spine: Subtle changes in sagittal spinal curves affect regional muscle activity. *Spine*, *34*(6), E208–E214.
5   Cortell-Tormo, J. M., García-Jaén, M., Chulvi-Medrano, I., Hernández-Sánchez, S., Lucas-Cuevas, Á. G., & Tortosa-Martínez, J. (2017). Influence of scapular position on the core musculature activation in the prone plank exercise. *Journal of Strength and Conditioning Research*, *31*(8), 2255–2262.
6   Kannan, P., Winser, S., Goonetilleke, R., & Cheing, G. (2019). Ankle positions potentially facilitating greater maximal contraction of pelvic floor muscles: A systematic review and meta-analysis. *Disability and Rehabilitation*, *41*(21), 2483–2491.
7   Campbell, A., Straker, L., O'Sullivan, P., Elliott, B., & Reid, M. (2013). Lumbar loading in the elite adolescent tennis serve: Link to low back pain. *Medical Science Sports Exercise*, *45*(8), 1562–1568.
8   De Carvalho, D., Grondin, D., & Callaghan, J. (2017). The impact of office chair features on lumbar lordosis, intervertebral joint and sacral tilt angles: A radiographic assessment. *Ergonomics*, *60*(10), 1393–1404.
9   Arjmand, N., & Shirazi-Adl, A. (2005). Biomechanics of changes in lumbar posture in static lifting. *Spine*, *30*(23), 2637–2648.
10 Jensen, G. M. (1980). Biomechanics of the lumbar intervertebral disk: A review. *Physical Therapy*, *60*(6), 765–773.
11 Coulter, D. (2004). *Anatomy of Hatha Yoga: A Manual for Students, Teachers, and Practitioners*. Honesdale, PA: Body and Breath.
12 Ko, M. J., Jung, E. J., Kim, M. H., & Oh, J. S. (2018). Effects of deep breathing on internal oblique and multifidus muscle activity in three sitting postures. *Journal of Physical Therapy Science*, *30*(4), 504–506.

13 Massery, M. (2006). Multisystem Consequences of Impaired Breathing Mechanics and/or Postural Control. In D. Frownfelter and E. Dean (eds.) *Cardiovascular and Pulmonary Physical Therapy Evidence and Practice*, 4th edition, pp. 695–717. St. Louis, MO: Elsevier Health Sciences.

14 Hodges, P. W., Eriksson, A., Shirley, D., & Gandevia, S. (2005). Intra-abdominal pressure increases stiffness of the lumbar spine. *Journal of Biomechanics, 38*(9), 1873–1880.

15 Hamaoui, A., Gonneau, E., & Le Bozec, S. (2010). Respiratory disturbance to posture varies according to the respiratory mode. *Neuroscience Letters, 475*(3), 141–144.

16 Massery, M., Hagins, M., Stafford, R., Moerchen, V., & Hodges, P. W. (2013). Effect of airway control by glottal structures on postural stability. *Journal of Applied Physiology, 115*(4), 483–490.

17 Frownfelter, D., Stevens, K., Massery, M., & Bernardoni, G. (2014). Do abdominal cutouts in thoracolumbosacral orthoses increase pulmonary function? *Clinical Orthopaedics and Related Research, 472*(2), 720–726.

18 Cheatham, M. L., De Waele, J. J., De Laet, I., De Keulenaer, B., et al. (2009). The impact of body position on intra-abdominal pressure measurement: A multicenter analysis. *Critical Care Medicine, 37*(7), 2187–2190.

19 Goldish, G. D., Quast, J. E., Blow, J. J., & Kuskowski, M. A. (1994). Postural effects on intra-abdominal pressure during Valsalva maneuver. *Archives of Physical Medicine and Rehabilitation, 75*(3), 324–327.

20 Lind, L. R., Lucente, V., & Kohn, N. (1996). Thoracic kyphosis and the prevalence of advanced uterine prolapse. *Obstetrics and Gynecology, 87*(4), 605–609.

21 Reeve, A., & Dilley, A. (2009). Effects of posture on the thickness of transversus abdominis in pain-free subjects. *Manual Therapy, 14*(6), 679–684.

22 Zafar, H., Albarrati, A., Alghadir, A. H., & Iqbal, Z. A. (2018). Effect of different head-neck postures on the respiratory function in healthy males. *Biomedical Research International*. doi: 10.1155/2018/4518269.

23 Smith, M. D., Russell, A., & Hodges, P. W. (2006). Disorders of breathing and continence have a stronger association with back pain than obesity and physical activity. *Australian Journal of Physiotherapy, 52*(1), 11–16.

24 Perri, M. A., & Halford, E. (2004). Pain and faulty breathing: A pilot study. *Journal of Bodywork and Movement Therapies, 8*(4), 297–306.

25 Perri, M. A., & Halford, E. (2004). Pain and faulty breathing: A pilot study. *Journal of Bodywork and Movement Therapies, 8*(4), 297–306.

26 Rathore, M., Trivedi, S., Abraham, J., & Sinha, M. B. (2017). Anatomical correlation of core muscle activation in different yogic postures. *International Journal of Yoga, 10*(2), 59–66.

27 Lauche, R., Wayne, P. M., Fehr, J., Stumpe, C., Dobos, G., & Cramer, H. (2017). Does postural awareness contribute to exercise-induced improvements in neck pain intensity? A secondary analysis of a randomized controlled trial evaluating Tai Chi and neck exercises. *Spine, 42*(16), 1195–1200.

28 Pelvic Guru (2019). Cervical, pelvic floor, and diaphragm connection: An interview with Susan Clinton. Accessed on March 6, 2022 at https://pelvicguru.com/cervical-pelvic-floor-and-diaphragm-connection-an-interview-with-susan-clinton.

29 Slater, D., Korakakis, V., O'Sullivan, P., Nolan, D., & O'Sullivan, K. (2019). "Sit up straight": Time to re-evaluate. *Journal of Orthopaedic and Sports Physical Therapy, 49*(8), 562–564.

30 Laird, R. A., Kent, P., & Keating, J. L. (2016). How consistent are lordosis, range of movement and lumbo-pelvic rhythm in people with and without back pain? *BioMed Central Musculoskeletal Disorders, 17*(1), 1–14.

31 Capson, A. C., Nashed, J., & Mclean, L. (2011). The role of lumbopelvic posture in pelvic floor muscle activation in continent women. *Journal of Electromyography and Kinesiology, 21*(1), 166–177.

32 Augeard, N., & Carroll, S. P. (2019). Core stability and low-back pain: A causal fallacy. *Journal of Exercise Rehabilitation, 15*(3), 493–495.

33 Kinetic Labs (2017, March 19). Perfect posture doesn't exist [Video file]. Accessed on August 7, 2022 at www.youtube.com/watch?v=cnLxcEMdjVk.

34 Sahrmann, S. A. (2002). Does postural assessment contribute to patient care? *Journal of Orthopaedic and Sports Physical Therapy, 32*(8), 376–379.

35 Sahrmann, S. A. (2002). Does postural assessment contribute to patient care? *Journal of Orthopaedic and Sports Physical Therapy, 32*(8), 376–379.

36 Harrison, D. E., Cailliet, R., Harrison, D. D., & Janik, T. J. (2002). How do anterior/posterior translations of the thoracic cage affect the sagittal lumbar spine, pelvic tilt, and thoracic kyphosis? *European Spine Journal, 11*(3), 287–293.

37 De Carvalho, D., Grondin, D., & Callaghan, J. (2017). The impact of office chair features on lumbar lordosis, intervertebral joint and sacral tilt angles: A radiographic assessment. *Ergonomics, 60*(10), 1393–1404.

38 Cook, G., Burton, L., Hoogenboom, B. J., & Voight, M. (2014). Functional movement screening: The use of fundamental movements as an assessment of function—Part 1. *International Journal of Sports and Physical Therapy, 9*(3), 396–409.

39 Cook, G., Burton, L., Hoogenboom, B. J., & Voight, M. (2014). Functional movement screening: The use of fundamental movements as an assessment of function—Part 2. *International Journal of Sports and Physical Therapy, 9*(4), 549–563.

40 Long, R. (2016). Lengthening the torso in yoga. Yoga U Online. Accessed on October 9, 2022 at www.yogauonline.com/yoga-anatomy/lengthening-torso-yoga-engaging-uddiyana-bandha-stabilize-spine-and-protect-low-back.

41 Johns Hopkins Medicine (2022). Muscle Pain: It May Actually Be Your Fascia. Accessed on September 8, 2022 at www.hopkinsmedicine.org/health/wellness-and-prevention/muscle-pain-it-may-actually-be-your-fascia.

42 Chapelle, S. L. (2016). Understanding and Approach to Treatment of Scars and Adhesions. In T. Liem, P. Tozzi, & A. Chila (eds.) *Fascia in the Osteopathic Field*, Chapter 51. London: Handspring Publications. p. 1.

43 Zügel, M., Maganaris, C. N., Wilke, J., Jurkat-Rott, K., et al. (2018). Fascial tissue research in sports medicine: From molecules to tissue adaptation, injury and diagnostics: Consensus statement. *British Journal of Sports Medicine, 52*(23), 1497.

44 Johns Hopkins Medicine (2022). Muscle Pain: It May Actually Be Your Fascia. Accessed on September 8, 2022 at www.hopkinsmedicine.org/health/wellness-and-prevention/muscle-pain-it-may-actually-be-your-fascia.

45 Bordoni, B., Lintonbon, D., & Morabito, B. (2018). Meaning of the solid and liquid fascia to reconsider the model of biotensegrity. *Cureus, 10*(7), e2922.

46 Myers, T. W. (2013). Anatomy Trains E-Book: *Myofascial Meridians for Manual and Movement Therapists*. Edinburgh: Livingstone Churchill.

47 Anatomy Trains (2022). A Brief History of Anatomy Trains. Accessed on September 21, 2022 at www.anatomytrains.com/about-us/history.

48 Zügel, M., Maganaris, C. N., Wilke, J., Jurkat-Rott, K., et al. (2018). Fascial tissue research in sports medicine: From molecules to tissue adaptation, injury and diagnostics: Consensus statement. *British Journal of Sports Medicine, 52*(23), 1497.

49 Pavan, P. G., Stecco, A., Stern, R., & Stecco, C. (2014). Painful connections: Densification versus fibrosis of fascia. *Current Pain and Headache Reports, 18*(8), 441.

50 Lee, D. (2008). Stability, continence and breathing—the role of fascia following pregnancy and delivery. *Journal of Bodywork and Movement Therapies, 12*, 333–348.

51 Masi, A. T., Nair, K., Evans, T., & Ghandour, Y. (2010). Clinical, biomechanical, and physiological translational interpretations of human resting myofascial tone or tension. *International Journal of Therapeutic Massage and Bodywork, 3*(4), 16–28.

52 Masi, A. T., Nair, K., Evans, T., & Ghandour, Y. (2010). Clinical, biomechanical, and physiological translational interpretations of human resting myofascial tone or tension. *International Journal of Therapeutic Massage and Bodywork, 3*(4), 16–28.

53 Masi, A. T., Nair, K., Evans, T., & Ghandour, Y. (2010). Clinical, biomechanical, and physiological translational interpretations of human resting myofascial tone or tension. *International Journal of Therapeutic Massage and Bodywork, 3*(4), 16–28.

54 Ingber, D. E. (2003). Tensegrity I. Cell structure and hierarchical systems biology. *Journal of Cell Science, 116*(7), 1157–1173.

55 Ingber, D. E. (2003). Tensegrity II. How structural networks influence cellular information processing networks. *Journal of Cell Science, 116*(8), 1397–1408.

56 Ingber, D. E., Wang, N., & Stamenović, D. (2015). Tensegrity, cellular biophysics, and the mechanics of living systems. *Reports on Progress in Physics, 77*(4), 046603.

57 Anatomy Trains (2022). A Brief History of Anatomy Trains. Accessed on September 21, 2022 at www.anatomytrains.com/about-us/history.

58 Beyond the Brick (2020, April 28). Physics teacher explains tensegrity sculptures with LEGO [Video file]. Accessed on February 13, 2022 at www.youtube.com/watch?v=xbHazHP3NI0.

Chapter 5

1 Akuthota, V., Ferreiro, A., Moore, T., & Fredericson, M. (2008). Core stability exercise principles. *Current Sports Medicine Reports, 7*(1), 39–44.

2 Nichols, T. R. (1994). A biomechanical perspective on spinal mechanisms of coordinated muscle activation. *Acta Anatomica, 15*, 1–13.

3 Kibler, W. B., Press, J., & Sciascia, A. (2006). The role of core stability in athletic function. *Sports Medicine, 36*(3), 189–198.

4 Du, W., Li, H., Omisore, O. M., Wang, L., Chen, W., & Sun, X. (2018). Co-contraction characteristics of lumbar muscles in patients with lumbar disc herniation during different types of movement. *BioMedical Engineering OnLine, 17*(1), 1–20.

5 McMullen, J., & Uhl, T. L. (2000). A kinetic chain approach for shoulder rehabilitation. *Journal of Athletic Training, 35*(3), 329–337.

6 Kibler, W. B., Press, J., & Sciascia, A. (2006). The role of core stability in athletic function. *Sports Medicine, 36*(3), 189–198.

7 Anderson, K., & Behm, D. G. (2005). Trunk muscle activity increases with unstable squat movements. *Canadian Journal of Applied Physiology, 30*(1), 33–45.

8 Chan, M. K., Chow, K. W., Lai, A. Y., Mak, N. K., Sze, J. C., & Tsang, S. M. (2017). The effects of therapeutic hip exercise with abdominal core activation on recruitment of the hip muscles. *BioMed Central Musculoskeletal Disorders, 18*(1), 313.

9 Rice, S. G. (2003). Using the kinetic chain theory in clinical practice. *Current Sports Medicine Reports, 2*, 289–290.

10 Key, J. (2013). "The core": Understanding it, and retraining its dysfunction. *Journal of Bodywork and Movement Therapies, 17*(4), 541–559.

11 Hodges, P. W., Sapsford, R., & Pengel, L. H. M. (2007). Postural and respiratory functions of the pelvic floor muscles. *Neurourology and Urodynamics: Official Journal of the International Continence Society, 26*(3), 362–371.

12 Hodges, P. W., & Richardson, C. A. (1997). Contraction of the abdominal muscles associated with movement of the lower limb. *Physical Therapy, 77*(2), 132–142.

13 Hodges, P. W., & Richardson, C. A. (1997). Feedforward contraction of transversus abdominis is not influenced by direction of arm movement. *Experimental Brain Research*, *114*(2), 362–370.

14 Moseley, G. L., Hodges, P. W., & Gandevia, S. C. (2002). Deep and superficial fibers of the lumbar multifidus muscle are differentially active during voluntary arm movements. *Spine*, *27*(2), E29–E36.

15 Hodges, P. W., & Gandevia, S. C. (2000). Activation of the human diaphragm during a repetitive postural task. *Journal of Physiology*, *522*(1), 165–175.

16 Hodges, P. W., & Gandevia, S. C. (2000). Changes in intra-abdominal pressure during postural and respiratory activation of the human diaphragm. *Journal of Applied Physiology*, *89*(3), 967–976.

17 McMullen, J., & Uhl, T. L. (2000). A kinetic chain approach for shoulder rehabilitation. *Journal of Athletic Training*, *35*(3), 329–337.

18 Massery, M. (2013, August 8). Glottal strategies—Massery PT—Mary Massery—If you can't breathe, you can't function [Video file]. Massery PT. Accessed on July 9, 2022 at www.youtube.com/watch?v=bF_uCPzYUDc.

19 Sjödahl, J., Kvist, J., Gutke, A., & Öberg, B. (2009). The postural response of the pelvic floor muscles during limb movements: A methodological electromyography study in parous women without lumbopelvic pain. *Clinical Biomechanics*, *24*(2), 183–189.

20 Bouisset, S., & Zattara, M. (1981). A sequence of postural movements precedes voluntary movement. *Neuroscience Letters*, *22*(3), 263–270.

21 Hodges, P. W., & Richardson, C. A. (1997). Feedforward contraction of transversus abdominis is not influenced by direction of arm movement. *Experimental Brain Research*, *114*(2), 362–370.

22 Hung, H. C., Hsiao, S. M., Chih, S. Y., Lin, H. H., & Tsauo, J. Y. (2010). An alternative intervention for urinary incontinence: Retraining diaphragmatic, deep abdominal and pelvic floor muscle coordinated function. *Manual Therapy*, *15*(3), 273–279.

23 Madill, S. J., Harvey, M. A., & McLean, L. (2010). Women with stress urinary incontinence demonstrate motor control differences during coughing. *Journal of Electromyography and Kinesiology*, *20*(5), 804–812.

24 Sapsford, R. R., Richardson, C. A., Maher, C. F., & Hodges, P. W. (2008). Pelvic floor muscle activity in different sitting postures in continent and incontinent women. *Archives of Physical Medicine and Rehabilitation*, *89*(9), 1741–1747.

25 Butrick, C. W. (2009). Pelvic floor hypertonic disorders: Identification and management. *Obstetrics and Gynecology Clinics*, *36*(3), 707–722.

26 O'Sullivan, P., Twomey, L., Allison, G., Sinclair, J., Miller, K., & Knox, J. (1997). Altered patterns of abdominal muscle activation in patients with chronic low back pain. *Australian Journal of Physiotherapy*, *43*(2), 91–98.

27 Smith, M. D., Coppieters, M. W., & Hodges, P. W. (2007). Postural activity of the pelvic floor muscles is delayed during rapid arm movements in women with stress urinary incontinence. *International Urogynecology Journal and Pelvic Floor Dysfunction*, *18*(8), 901–911.

28 Hodges, P. W., & Richardson, C. A. (1996). Inefficient muscular stabilization of the lumbar spine associated with low back pain: A motor control evaluation of transversus abdominis. *Spine*, *21*(22), 2640–2650.

29 O'Sullivan, P., Twomey, L., Allison, G., Sinclair, J., Miller, K., & Knox, J. (1997). Altered patterns of abdominal muscle activation in patients with chronic low back pain. *Australian Journal of Physiotherapy*, *43*(2), 91–98.

30 McCook, D. T., Vicenzino, B., & Hodges, P. W. (2009). Activity of deep abdominal muscles increases during submaximal flexion and extension efforts but antagonist

co-contraction remains unchanged. *Journal of Electromyography and Kinesiology*, *19*(5), 754–762.

31 Lederman, E. (2010). The myth of core stability. *Journal of Bodywork and Movement Therapies*, *14*(1), 84–98.

32 Augeard, N., & Carroll, S. P. (2019). Core stability and low-back pain: A causal fallacy. *Journal of Exercise Rehabilitation*, *15*(3), 493–495.

33 Smith, B. E., Littlewood, C., & May, S. (2014). An update of stabilisation exercises for low back pain: A systematic review with meta-analysis. *BioMed Central Musculoskeletal Disorders*, *15*(1), 1–21.

34 Lederman, E. (2010). The myth of core stability. *Journal of Bodywork and Movement Therapies*, *14*(1), 84–98.

35 Reeves, N. P., Cholewicki, J., Van Dieën, J. H., Kawchuk, G., & Hodges, P. W. (2019). Are stability and instability relevant concepts for back pain? *Journal of Orthopaedic and Sports Physical Therapy*, *49*(6), 415–424.

36 Reeves, N. P., Cholewicki, J., Van Dieën, J. H., Kawchuk, G., & Hodges, P. W. (2019). Are stability and instability relevant concepts for back pain? *Journal of Orthopaedic and Sports Physical Therapy*, *49*(6), 415–424.

37 Sullivan, M. (2018, December 17) Diaphragm, breath and bandhas: Yoga for core stability and integration—Session 1 [Training course].

38 Hung, H. C., Hsiao, S. M., Chih, S. Y., Lin, H. H., & Tsauo, J. Y. (2010). An alternative intervention for urinary incontinence: Retraining diaphragmatic, deep abdominal and pelvic floor muscle coordinated function. *Manual Therapy*, *15*(3), 273–279.

39 Ashton-Miller, J. A., & DeLancey, J. (2007). Functional anatomy of the female pelvic floor. *Annals of the New York Academy of Sciences*, *1101*(1), 266–296.

40 Sapsford, R. (2004). Rehabilitation of pelvic floor muscles utilizing trunk stabilization. *Manual Therapy*, *9*(1), 3–12.

41 Ashton-Miller, J. A., & DeLancey, J. (2007). Functional anatomy of the female pelvic floor. *Annals of the New York Academy of Sciences*, *1101*(1), 266–296.

42 Raizada, V., & Mittal, R. K. (2008). Pelvic floor anatomy and applied physiology. *Gastroenterology Clinics of North America*, *37*(3), 493–509.

43 Raizada, V., & Mittal, R. K. (2008). Pelvic floor anatomy and applied physiology. *Gastroenterology Clinics of North America*, *37*(3), 493–509.

44 Sapsford, R. (2004). Rehabilitation of pelvic floor muscles utilizing trunk stabilization. *Manual Therapy*, *9*(1), 3–12.

45 DeLancey, J. O. (1996). Stress urinary incontinence: Where are we now, where should we go? *American Journal of Obstetrics and Gynecology*, *175*(2), 311–319.

46 Hodges, P. W., Sapsford, R., & Pengel, L. H. M. (2007). Postural and respiratory functions of the pelvic floor muscles. *Neurourology and Urodynamics: Official Journal of the International Continence Society*, *26*(3), 362–371.

47 Smith, M. D., Coppieters, M. W., & Hodges, P. W. (2007). Postural activity of the pelvic floor muscles is delayed during rapid arm movements in women with stress urinary incontinence. *International Urogynecological Journal of Pelvic Floor Dysfunction*, *18*(8), 901–911.

48 Sjödahl, J., Kvist, J., Gutke, A., & Öberg, B. (2009). The postural response of the pelvic floor muscles during limb movements: A methodological electromyography study in parous women without lumbopelvic pain. *Clinical Biomechanics*, *24*(2), 183–189.

49 Hjartardóttir, S., Nilsson, J., Petersen, C., & Lingman, G. (1997). The female pelvic floor: A dome—not a basin. *Acta Obstetricia et Gynecologica Scandinavica*, *76*(6), 567–571.

50 Gordon, K. E., & Reed, O. (2020). The role of the pelvic floor in respiration: A multidisciplinary literature review. *Journal of Voice*, *34*(2), 243–249.

51 Hodges, P. W., Sapsford, R., & Pengel, L. H. M. (2007). Postural and respiratory functions of the pelvic floor muscles. *Neurourology and Urodynamics: Official Journal of the International Continence Society*, *26*(3), 362–371.

52 Kitani, L. J., Apte, G. G., Dedrick, G. S., Sizer, P. S., & Brismée, J. M. (2014). Effect of variations in forced expiration effort on pelvic floor activation in asymptomatic women. *Journal of Women's Health Physical Therapy*, *38*(1), 19–27.

53 Aljuraifani, R., Stafford, R. E., Hall, L. M., van den Hoorn, W., & Hodges, P. W. (2019). Task-specific differences in respiration-related activation of deep and superficial pelvic floor muscles. *Journal of Applied Physiology*, *126*(5), 1343–1351.

54 Prosko, S. (2021). Yoga Therapy: An Evidence-Informed Integrative Approach to Help People Enhance Pelvic Floor Health (Trainer Manual). PhysioYoga. Course available at https://physioyoga.ca/yoga-therapy-an-evidence-informed-integrative-approach-to-help-people-enhance-pelvic-floor-health, accessed on January 4, 2023.

55 Moalli, P. A., Jones, I. S., Meyn, L. A., & Zyczynski, H. M. (2003). Risk factors associated with pelvic floor disorders in women undergoing surgical repair. *Obstetrics and Gynecology*, *101*, 869–874.

56 Sultan, A. H., Kamm, M. A., & Hudson, C. N. (1994). Pudendal nerve damage during labour: Prospective study before and after childbirth. *British Journal of Obstetrics and Gynecology*, *101*, 22–28.

57 Nichols, C. M., Gill, E. J., Nguyen, T., Barber, M. D., & Hurt, W. G. (2004). Anal sphincter injury in women with pelvic floor disorders. *Obstetrics and Gynecology*, *104*, 690–696.

58 Dietz, H. P., & Schierlitz, L. (2005). Pelvic floor trauma in childbirth—myth or reality? *Australian and New Zealand Journal of Obstetrics and Gynaecology*, *45*, 3–11.

59 Bhattacherjee, A., Rumi, M. A., Staecker, H., & Smith, P. G. (2013). Bone morphogenetic protein 4 mediates estrogen-regulated sensory axon plasticity in the adult female reproductive tract. *Journal of Neuroscience*, *33*, 1050–1061a.

60 Blakeman, P. J., Hilton, P., & Bulmer, J. N. (2001). Cellular proliferation in the female lower urinary tract with reference to oestrogen status. *British Journal of Obstetrics and Gynecology*, *108*, 813–816.

61 Lee, J. H., & Lee, S. W. (2016). Testosterone and chronic prostatitis/chronic pelvic pain syndrome: A propensity score-matched analysis. *Journal of Sex Medicine*, *13*, 1047–1055.

62 Laumann, E. O., Paik, A., & Rosen, R. C. (1999). Sexual dysfunction in the United States: Prevalence and predictors. *JAMA*, *281*, 537–544.

63 Both, S., Van Lunsen, R., Weijenborg, P., & Laan, E. (2012). A new device for simultaneous measurement of pelvic floor muscle activity and vaginal blood flow. *Journal of Sex Medicine*, *9*, 2888–2902.

64 Bogner, H. R., O'Donnell, A. J., de Vries, H. F., Northington, G. M., & Joo, J. H. (2011). The temporal relationship between anxiety disorders and urinary incontinence among community-dwelling adults. *Journal of Anxiety Disorders*, *25*, 203–208.

65 Felde, G., Bjelland, I., & Hunskaar, S. (2012). Anxiety and depression associated with incontinence in middle-aged women: A large Norwegian cross-sectional study. *International Urogynecology Journal*, *23*, 299–306.

66 Vrijens, D., Berghmans, B., Nieman, F., van Os, J., & van Koeveringe, G. (2017). Prevalence of anxiety and depressive symptoms and their association with pelvic floor dysfunctions—A cross-sectional cohort study at a pelvic care centre. *Neurourology Urodynamics*, *36*, 1816–1823.

67 Vrijens, D. M. J., Drossaerts, J. M. A. F. L., Rademakers, K., Smit, M., et al. (2017). Associations of psychometric affective parameters with urodynamic investigation for urinary frequency. *Lower Urinary Tract Symptoms*, *9*, 166–170.

68 Zilberlicht, A., Haya, N., Feferkorn, I., Goldschmidt, E., Kaldawy, A., & Abramov, Y. (2018). Somatic, psychological, and sexual triggers for overactive bladder syndrome in women. *Neurourology and Urodynamics: Official Journal of the International Continence Society, 37*(1), 163–168.

69 Prosko, S. (2021). Yoga Therapy: An Evidence-Informed Integrative Approach to Help People Enhance Pelvic Floor Health (Trainer Manual). PhysioYoga. Course available at https://physioyoga.ca/yoga-therapy-an-evidence-informed-integrative-approach-to-help-people-enhance-pelvic-floor-health, accessed on January 4, 2023.

70 Sapsford, R. R., Richardson, C. A., Maher, C. F., & Hodges, P. W. (2008). Pelvic floor muscle activity in different sitting postures in continent and incontinent women. *Archives of Physical Medicine and Rehabilitation, 89*, 1741–1747.

71 Halski, T., Ptaszkowski, K., Słupska, L., Dymarek, R., & Paprocka-Borowicz, M. (2017). Relationship between lower limb position and pelvic floor muscle surface electromyography activity in menopausal women: A prospective observational study. *Clinical Interventions in Aging, 12*, 75–83.

72 Capson, A. C., Nashed, J., & Mclean, L. (2011). The role of lumbopelvic posture in pelvic floor muscle activation in continent women. *Journal of Electromyography and Kinesiology, 21*, 166–177.

73 Study.com (2022). Length-Tension Relationship in Skeletal Muscle [Video file]. Accessed on February 19, 2022 at https://study.com/academy/lesson/length-tension-relationship-in-skeletal-muscle.html.

74 Sapsford, R. R., Richardson, C. A., & Stanton, W. R. (2006). Sitting posture affects pelvic floor muscle activity in parous women: An observational study. *Australian Journal of Physiotherapy, 52*, 219–222.

75 Sapsford, R. R., Richardson, C. A., Maher, C. F., & Hodges, P. W. (2008). Pelvic floor muscle activity in different sitting postures in continent and incontinent women. *Archives of Physical Medicine and Rehabilitation, 89*(9), 1741–1747.

76 Capson, A. C., Nashed, J., & Mclean, L. (2011). The role of lumbopelvic posture in pelvic floor muscle activation in continent women. *Journal of Electromyography and Kinesiology, 21*(1), 166–177.

77 Capson, A. C., Nashed, J., & Mclean, L. (2011). The role of lumbopelvic posture in pelvic floor muscle activation in continent women. *Journal of Electromyography and Kinesiology, 21*(1), 166–177.

78 Butrick, C. W. (2009). Pelvic floor hypertonic disorders: Identification and management. *Obstetrics and Gynecology Clinics, 36*(3), 707–722.

79 Butrick, C. W. (2009). Pelvic floor hypertonic disorders: Identification and management. *Obstetrics and Gynecology Clinics, 36*(3), 707–722.

80 Dufour, S., Vandyken, B., Forget, M. J., & Vandyken, C. (2018). Association between lumbopelvic pain and pelvic floor dysfunction in women: A cross sectional study. *Musculoskeletal Science and Practice, 34*, 47–53.

81 Tu, F. F., As-Sanie, S., & Steege, J. F. (2005). Musculoskeletal causes of chronic pelvic pain: A systematic review of existing therapies: Part II. *Obstetrical and Gynecological Survey, 60*(7), 474–483.

82 Haugstad, G. K., Haugstad, T. S., Kirste, U. M., Leganger, S., et al. (2006). Posture, movement patterns, and body awareness in women with chronic pelvic pain. *Journal of Psychosomatic Research, 61*(5), 637–644.

83 Huang, W. C., & Yang, J. M. (2018). Menopause is associated with impaired responsiveness of involuntary pelvic floor muscle contractions to sudden intra-abdominal pressure rise in women with pelvic floor symptoms: A retrospective study. *Neurourology and Urodynamics: Official Journal of the International Continence Society, 37*(3), 1128–1136.

84 Nygaard, I. E., Thompson, F. L., Svengalis, S. L., & Albright, J. P. (1994). Urinary incontinence in elite nulliparous athletes. *Obstetrics and Gynecology, 84*(2), 183–187.

85 Butrick, C. W. (2009). Pelvic floor hypertonic disorders: Identification and management. *Obstetrics and Gynecology Clinics, 36*(3), 707–722.

86 Hung, H. C., Hsiao, S. M., Chih, S. Y., Lin, H. H., & Tsauo, J. Y. (2010). An alternative intervention for urinary incontinence: Retraining diaphragmatic, deep abdominal and pelvic floor muscle coordinated function. *Manual Therapy, 15*(3), 273–279.

87 Kim, H., Suzuki, T., Yoshida, Y., & Yoshida, H. (2007). Effectiveness of multidimensional exercises for the treatment of stress urinary incontinence in elderly community-dwelling Japanese women: A randomized, controlled, crossover trial. *Journal of the American Geriatric Society, 55,* 1932–1939.

88 Barbato, K. A., Wiebe, J. W., Cline, T. W., & Hellier, S. D. (2014). Web-based treatment for women with stress urinary incontinence. *International Journal of Urological Nursing, 34,* 252–257.

89 Lee, D., & Lee, L.-J. (2004, November). *Stress Urinary Incontinence—A Consequence of Failed Load Transfer Through the Pelvis?* Presented at the 5th World Interdisciplinary Conference on Low Back and Pelvic Pain, Melbourne, Australia.

90 Baker, J., Costa, D., & Nygaard, I. (2012). Mindfulness-based stress reduction for treatment of urinary urge incontinence: A pilot study. *Female Pelvic Medical Reconstructive Surgery, 18,* 46–49.

91 Dugan, S. A., Lavender, M. D., Hebert-Beirne, J., & Brubaker, L. (2013). A pelvic floor fitness program for older women with urinary symptoms: A feasibility study. *American Journal of Physical Medicine and Rehabilitation, 5,* 672–676.

92 Huang, A. J., Chesney, M. A., Schembri, M., & Subak, L. L. (2018). PD32-01 a randomized trial of a group-based therapeutic yoga program for ambulatory women with urinary incontinence. *Journal of Urology, 199*(4), e645.

93 Hwang, U. J., Lee, M. S., Jung, S. H., Ahn, S. H., & Kwon, O. Y. (2021). Relationship between sexual function and pelvic floor and hip muscle strength in women with stress urinary incontinence. *Journal of Sex Medicine, 9*(2), 100317.

94 Foster, S. N., Spitznagle, T. M., Tuttle, L. J., Sutcliffe, S., et al. (2021). Hip and pelvic floor muscle strength in women with and without urgency and frequency—predominant lower urinary tract symptoms. *Journal of Women's Health Physical Therapy, 45*(3), 126–134.

95 Howard, L. (2017). *Pelvic Liberation: Using Yoga, Self-Inquiry, and Breath Awareness for Pelvic Health,* 1st edition. Emeryville, CA: Leslie Howard Yoga.

96 Junginger, B., Seibt, E., & Baessler, K. (2014). Bladder-neck effective, integrative pelvic floor rehabilitation program: Follow-up investigation. *European Journal of Obstetrics and Gynecology and Reproductive Biology, 174,* 150–153.

97 Madill, S. J., Harvey, M. A., & McLean, L. (2010). Women with stress urinary incontinence demonstrate motor control differences during coughing. *Journal of Electromyography and Kinesiology, 20*(5), 804–812.

98 Madill, S. J., Harvey, M. A., & McLean, L. (2010). Women with stress urinary incontinence demonstrate motor control differences during coughing. *Journal of Electromyography and Kinesiology, 20*(5), 804–812.

99 Smith, M. D., Coppieters, M. W., & Hodges, P. W. (2008). Is balance different in women with and without stress urinary incontinence? *Neurourology and Urodynamics: Official Journal of the International Continence Society, 27*(1), 71–78.

100 Aljuraifani, R., Stafford, R. E., Hall, L. M., van den Hoorn, W., & Hodges, P. W. (2019). Task-specific differences in respiration-related activation of deep and superficial pelvic floor muscles. *Journal of Applied Physiology, 126*(5), 1343–1351.

101 Talasz, H., Kremser, C., Kofler, M., Kalchschmid, E., Lechleitner, M, & Rudisch, A. (2011). Phase-locked parallel movement of diaphragm and pelvic floor during

breathing and coughing—A dynamic MRI investigation in healthy females. *International Urogynecology Journal, 22*(1), 61–68.

102 Sjödahl, J., Kvist, J., Gutke, A., & Öberg, B. (2009). The postural response of the pelvic floor muscles during limb movements: A methodological electromyography study in parous women without lumbopelvic pain. *Clinical Biomechanics, 24*(2), 183–189.

103 Bordoni, B., & Zanier, E. (2013). Anatomical connections of the diaphragm: Influence of respiration on the body system. *Journal of Multidisciplinary Healthcare, 6*, 281–291.

104 Dugan, S. A., Lavender, M. D., Hebert-Beirne, J., & Brubaker, L. (2013). A pelvic floor fitness program for older women with urinary symptoms: A feasibility study. *American Journal of Physical Medicine and Rehabilitation, 5*, 672–676.

105 Foster, S. N., Spitznagle, T. M., Tuttle, L. J., Sutcliffe, S., et al. (2021). Hip and pelvic floor muscle strength in women with and without urgency and frequency—predominant lower urinary tract symptoms. *Journal of Women's Health Physical Therapy, 45*(3), 126–134.

106 Bo, K. (2004). Pelvic floor muscle training is effective in treatment of female stress urinary incontinence, but how does it work? *International Urogynecological Journal of Pelvic Floor Dysfunction, 2*, 76–84.

107 Bo, K. (2004). Pelvic floor muscle training is effective in treatment of female stress urinary incontinence, but how does it work? *International Urogynecological Journal of Pelvic Floor Dysfunction, 2*, 76–84.

108 Bo, K. (2004). Pelvic floor muscle training is effective in treatment of female stress urinary incontinence, but how does it work? *International Urogynecological Journal of Pelvic Floor Dysfunction, 2*, 76–84.

109 Hanno, P. M., Erickson, D., Moldwin, R., Faraday, M. M., & American Urological Association (2015). Diagnosis and treatment of interstitial cystitis/bladder pain syndrome: AUA guideline amendment. *Journal of Urology, 193*, 1545–1553.

110 Hung, H. C., Hsiao, S. M., Chih, S. Y., Lin, H. H., & Tsauo, J. Y. (2010). An alternative intervention for urinary incontinence: Retraining diaphragmatic, deep abdominal and pelvic floor muscle coordinated function. *Manual Therapy, 15*, 273–279.

111 Kim, H., Suzuki, T., Yoshida, Y., & Yoshida, H. (2007). Effectiveness of multidimensional exercises for the treatment of stress urinary incontinence in elderly community-dwelling Japanese women: A randomized, controlled, crossover trial. *Journal of the American Geriatric Society, 55*, 1932–1939.

112 Barbato, K. A., Wiebe, J. W., Cline, T. W., & Hellier, S. D. (2014). Web-based treatment for women with stress urinary incontinence. *International Journal of Urological Nursing, 34*, 252–257.

113 Lee, D., & Lee, L.-J. (2004, November). *Stress Urinary Incontinence—A Consequence of Failed Load Transfer Through the Pelvis?* Presented at the 5th World Interdisciplinary Conference on Low Back and Pelvic Pain, Melbourne, Australia.

114 Baker, J., Costa, D., & Nygaard, I. (2012). Mindfulness-based stress reduction for treatment of urinary urge incontinence: A pilot study. *Female Pelvic Medical Reconstructive Surgery, 18*, 46–49.

115 Dugan, S. A., Lavender, M. D., Hebert-Beirne, J., & Brubaker, L. (2013). A pelvic floor fitness program for older women with urinary symptoms: A feasibility study. *American Journal of Physical Medicine and Rehabilitation, 5*, 672–676.

116 Huang, A. J., Chesney, M. A., Schembri, M., & Subak, L. L. (2018). PD32–01 a randomized trial of a group-based therapeutic yoga program for ambulatory women with urinary incontinence. *Journal of Urology, 199*(4), e645.

117 Hwang, U. J., Lee, M. S., Jung, S. H., Ahn, S. H., & Kwon, O. Y. (2021). Relationship between sexual function and pelvic floor and hip muscle strength in women with stress urinary incontinence. *Journal of Sex Medicine*, *9*(2), 100317.

118 Foster, S. N., Spitznagle, T. M., Tuttle, L. J., Sutcliffe, S., et al. (2021). Hip and pelvic floor muscle strength in women with and without urgency and frequency— predominant lower urinary tract symptoms. *Journal of Women's Health Physical Therapy*, *45*(3), 126–134.

119 Dumoulin, C., Cacciari, L. P., & Hay-Smith, E. J. C. (2018). Pelvic floor muscle training versus no treatment, or inactive control treatments, for urinary incontinence in women. *Cochrane Database of Systematic Reviews*, *10*, CD005654.

120 Butrick, C. W. (2009). Pelvic floor hypertonic disorders: Identification and management. *Obstetrics and Gynecology Clinics*, *36*(3), 707–722.

121 Lamin, E., Parrillo, L. M., Newman, D. K., & Smith, A. L. (2016). Pelvic floor muscle training: Underutilization in the USA. *Current Urology Reports*, *17*(2), 1–7.

122 Tu, F. F., As-Sanie, S., & Steege, J. F. (2005). Musculoskeletal causes of chronic pelvic pain: A systematic review of existing therapies: part II. *Obstetrical & Gynecological Survey*, *60*(7), 474–483.

123 Madill, S. J., & McLean, L. (2008). Quantification of abdominal and pelvic floor muscle synergies in response to voluntary pelvic floor muscle contractions. *Journal of Electromyography and Kinesiology*, *18*(6), 955–964.

124 Hung, H. C., Hsiao, S. M., Chih, S. Y., Lin, H. H., & Tsauo, J. Y. (2010). An alternative intervention for urinary incontinence: Retraining diaphragmatic, deep abdominal and pelvic floor muscle coordinated function. *Manual Therapy*, *15*(3), 273–279.

125 Junginger, B., Seibt, E., & Baessler, K. (2014). Bladder-neck effective, integrative pelvic floor rehabilitation program: Follow-up investigation. *European Journal of Obstetrics and Gynecology and Reproductive Biology*, *174*, 150–153.

126 Sapsford, R. R., Hodges, P. W., Richardson, C. A., Cooper, D. H., Markwell, S. J., & Jull, G. A. (2001). Co-activation of the abdominal and pelvic floor muscles during voluntary exercises. *Neurourology and Urodynamics: Official Journal of the International Continence Society*, *20*(1), 31–42.

127 Neumann, P., & Gill, V. (2002). Pelvic floor and abdominal muscle interaction: EMG activity and intra-abdominal pressure. *International Urogynecology Journal*, *13*(2), 125–132.

128 Hung, H. C., Hsiao, S. M., Chih, S. Y., Lin, H. H., & Tsauo, J. Y. (2010). An alternative intervention for urinary incontinence: Retraining diaphragmatic, deep abdominal and pelvic floor muscle coordinated function. *Manual Therapy*, *15*(3), 273–279.

129 Neumann, P., & Gill, V. (2002). Pelvic floor and abdominal muscle interaction: EMG activity and intra-abdominal pressure. *International Urogynecology Journal*, *13*(2), 125–132.

130 Bo, K. (2004). Pelvic floor muscle training is effective in treatment of female stress urinary incontinence, but how does it work? *International Urogynecology Journal*, *2*, 76–84.

131 Lasak, A. M., Jean-Michel, M., Le, P. U., Durgam, R., & Harroche, J. (2018). The role of pelvic floor muscle training in the conservative and surgical management of female stress urinary incontinence: Does the strength of the pelvic floor muscles matter? *American Journal of Physical Medicine & Rehabilitation*, *10*(11), 1198–1210.

132 Hodges, P. W. (1999). Is there a role for transversus abdominis in lumbo-pelvic stability? *Manual Therapy*, *4*(2), 74–86.

133 Sapsford, R. R., Hodges, P. W., Richardson, C. A., Cooper, D. H., Markwell, S. J., & Jull, G. A. (2001). Co-activation of the abdominal and pelvic floor muscles during voluntary exercises. *Neurourology and Urodynamics: Official Journal of the International Continence Society*, *20*(1), 31–42.

134 Cholewicki, J., Juluru, K., & McGill, S. M. (1999). Intra-abdominal pressure mechanism for stabilizing the lumbar spine. *Journal of Biomechanics, 32*(1), 13–17.

135 Hides, J., Wilson, S., Stanton, W., McMahon, S., et al. (2006). An MRI investigation into the function of the transversus abdominis muscle during "drawing-in" of the abdominal wall. *Spine, 31*(6), E175–E178.

136 Hodges, P. W. (1999). Is there a role for transversus abdominis in lumbo-pelvic stability? *Manual Therapy, 4*(2), 74–86.

137 Urquhart, D. M., Barker, P. J., Hodges, P. W., Story, I. H., & Briggs, C. A. (2005). Regional morphology of the transversus abdominis and obliquus internus and externus abdominis muscles. *Clinical Biomechanics, 20*(3), 233–241.

138 Rathore et al. (2017), citing Richardson, C., Jull, G., Toppenberg, R., & Comerford, M. (1992). Techniques for active lumbar stabilisation for spinal protection: A pilot study. *Australian Journal of Physiotherapy, 38*, 105–112.

139 Hodges, P. W., & Richardson, C. A. (1999). Transversus abdominis and superficial abdominal muscles are controlled independently in a postural task. *Neuroscience Letters, 265*(2), 91–94.

140 Hodges, P. W., & Richardson, C. A. (1997). Feedforward contraction of transversus abdominis is not influenced by direction of arm movement. *Experimental Brain Research, 114*(2), 362–370.

141 Cresswell, A. G., Oddsson, L., & Thorstensson, A. (1994). The influence of sudden perturbations on trunk muscle activity and intra-abdominal pressure while standing. *Experimental Brain Research, 98*, 336–341.

142 Hodges, P. W., Sapsford, R., & Pengel, L. H. M. (2007). Postural and respiratory functions of the pelvic floor muscles. *Neurourology and Urodynamics: Official Journal of the International Continence Society, 26*(3), 362–371.

143 Hodges, P. W., & Richardson, C. A. (1999). Transversus abdominis and superficial abdominal muscles are controlled independently in a postural task. *Neuroscience Letters, 265*(2), 91–94.

144 McCook, D. T., Vicenzino, B., & Hodges, P. W. (2009). Activity of deep abdominal muscles increases during submaximal flexion and extension efforts but antagonist co-contraction remains unchanged. *Journal of Electromyography and Kinesiology, 19*(5), 754–762.

145 Hodges, P. W., & Richardson, C. A. (1999). Transversus abdominis and the superficial abdominal muscles are controlled independently in a postural task. *Neuroscience Letters, 265*(2), 91–94.

146 McGill, S. M., Grenier, S., Kavcic, N., & Cholewicki, J. (2003). Coordination of muscle activity to assure stability of the lumbar spine. *Journal of Electromyography and Kinesiology, 13*(4), 353–359.

147 Hodges, P. W. (1999). Is there a role for transversus abdominis in lumbo-pelvic stability? *Manual Therapy, 4*(2), 74–86.

148 Hodges, P. W., & Richardson, C. A. (1999). Transversus abdominis and the superficial abdominal muscles are controlled independently in a postural task. *Neuroscience Letters, 265*(2), 91–94.

149 Bartelink, D. L. (1957). The role of abdominal pressure in relieving the pressure on the lumbar intervertebral discs. *Journal of Bone and Joint Surgery. British Volume, 39B*(4), 718–725.

150 Chan, E. W. M., Hamid, M. S. A., Nadzalan, A. M., & Hafiz, E. (2020). Abdominal muscle activation: An EMG study of the Sahrmann five-level core stability test. *Hong Kong Physiotherapy Journal, 40*(2), 89–97.

151 Hodges, P. W., & Richardson, C. A. (1996). Inefficient muscular stabilization of the lumbar spine associated with low back pain: A motor control evaluation of transversus abdominis. *Spine, 21*(22), 2640–2650.

152 Hodges, P. W., & Richardson, C. A. (1998). Delayed postural contraction of trans-versus abdominis in low back pain associated with movement of the lower limb. *Journal of Spine Disorders*, *11*(1), 46–56.

153 Hodges, P. W., & Richardson, C. A. (1999). Altered trunk muscle recruitment in people with low back pain with upper limb movement at different speeds. *Archives of Physical Medicine and Rehabilitation*, *80*(9), 1005–1012.

154 Hodges, P. W. (2000). The role of the motor system in spinal pain: Implications for rehabilitation of the athlete following low back pain. *Journal of Science and Medicine in Sport*, *3*(3), 243–253.

155 Hodges, P. W., van den Hoorn, W., Dawson, A., & Cholewicki, J. (2009). Changes in the mechanical properties of the trunk in low back pain may be associated with recurrence. *Journal of Biomechanics*, *42*(1), 61–66.

156 Hodges, P. W. (2001). Changes in motor planning of feedforward postural responses of the trunk muscles in low back pain. *Experimental Brain Research*, *141*(2), 261–266.

157 Hodges, P. W. (2003). Core stability exercise in chronic low back pain. *Orthopedic Clinics of North America*, *34*, 245–254.

158 O'Sullivan, P., Twomey, L., Allison, G., Sinclair, J., Miller, K., & Knox, J. (1997). Altered patterns of abdominal muscle activation in patients with chronic low back pain. *Australian Journal of Physiotherapy*, *43*(2), 91–98.

159 Hodges, P. W. (1999). Is there a role for transversus abdominis in lumbo-pelvic stability? *Manual Therapy*, *4*(2), 74–86.

160 Hides, J., Wilson, S., Stanton, W., McMahon, S., et al. (2006). An MRI investigation into the function of the transversus abdominis muscle during "drawing-in" of the abdominal wall. *Spine*, *31*(6), E175–E178.

161 Thompson, J. A., O'Sullivan, P. B., Briffa, N. K., & Neumann, P. (2006). Differences in muscle activation patterns during pelvic floor muscle contraction and valsalva manoeuvre. *Neurourology and Urodynamics: Official Journal of the International Continence Society*, *25*(2), 148–155.

162 Pinto, R. Z., Ferreira, P. H., Franco, M. R., Ferreira, M. C., et al. (2011). The effect of lumbar posture on abdominal muscle thickness during an isometric leg task in people with and without non-specific low back pain. *Manual Therapy*, *16*(6), 578–584.

163 Kujala et al. (1992), cited in Gildea, J. E., Hides, J. A., & Hodges, P. W. (2014). Morphology of the abdominal muscles in ballet dancers with and without low back pain: A magnetic resonance imaging study. *Journal of Science and Medicine in Sports*, *17*(5), 452–456.

164 Kujala et al. (1994), cited in Gildea, J. E., Hides, J. A., & Hodges, P. W. (2014). Morphology of the abdominal muscles in ballet dancers with and without low back pain: A magnetic resonance imaging study. *Journal of Science and Medicine in Sports*, *17*(5), 452–456.

165 Rowley, K. M., Smith, J. A., & Kulig, K. (2019). Reduced trunk coupling in persons with recurrent low back pain is associated with greater deep-to-superficial trunk muscle activation ratios during the balance-dexterity task. *Journal of Orthopaedic and Sports Physical Therapy*, *49*(12), 887–898.

166 van der Hulst, M., Vollenbroek-Hutten, M. M., Rietman, J. S., & Hermens, H. J. (2010). Lumbar and abdominal muscle activity during walking in subjects with chronic low back pain: Support of the "guarding" hypothesis? *Journal of Electromyography and Kinesiology*, *20*(1), 31–38.

167 Schinkel-Ivy, A., Nairn, B. C., & Drake, J. D. (2013). Investigation of trunk muscle co-contraction and its association with low back pain development during prolonged sitting. *Journal of Electromyography and Kinesiology*, *23*(4), 778–786.

168 Dufour, S., & Brittal, S. (2018). Pregnancy-related pelvic girdle pain: Embrace the evidence and move beyond biomechanics. *Journal of Yoga and Physiology*, *3*(5), 555–562.

169 Allison, G. T., & Morris, S. L. (2008). Transversus abdominis and core stability: Has the pendulum swung? *British Journal of Sports Medicine*, *42*(11), 930–931.

170 Allison, G. T., & Morris, S. L. (2008). Transversus abdominis and core stability: Has the pendulum swung? *British Journal of Sports Medicine*, *42*(11), 930–931.

171 Schinkel-Ivy, A., Nairn, B. C., & Drake, J. D. (2013). Investigation of trunk muscle co-contraction and its association with low back pain development during prolonged sitting. *Journal of Electromyography and Kinesiology*, *23*(4), 778–786.

172 Hudani, M. (2022). *Diastasis Rectus Abdominis: A New Era—A Guide for Health and Fitness Professionals*. Peace River, Alberta: Munira Hudani PT Inc. p. 2.

173 Gluppe, S. L., Hilde, G., Tennfjord, M. K., Engh, M. E., & Bø, K. (2018). Effect of a postpartum training program on the prevalence of diastasis recti abdominis in postpartum primiparous women: A randomized controlled trial. *Physical Therapy*, *98*(4), 260–268.

174 Tuttle, L. J., Fasching, J., Keller, A., Patel, M., et al. (2018). Noninvasive treatment of postpartum diastasis recti abdominis: A pilot study. *Journal of Women's Health Physical Therapy*, *42*(2), 65–75.

175 Mota, P. G., Pascoal, A. G., Carita, A. I., & Bø, K. (2015). The immediate effects on inter-rectus distance of abdominal crunch and drawing-in exercises during pregnancy and the postpartum period. *Journal of Orthopaedic and Sports Physical Therapy*, *45*(10), 781–788.

176 Sancho, M. F., Pascoal, A. G., Mota, P., & Bø, K. (2015). Abdominal exercises affect inter-rectus distance in postpartum women: A two-dimensional ultrasound study. *Physiotherapy*, *101*(3), 286–291.

177 Arranz-Martín, B., Navarro-Brazález, B., Sánchez-Sánchez, B., McLean, L., Carazo-Díaz, C., & Torres-Lacomba, M. (2022). The impact of hypopressive abdominal exercise on linea alba morphology in women who are postpartum: A short-term cross-sectional study. *Physical Therapy*, *102*(8), pzac086.

178 Hudani, M. (2022). *Diastasis Rectus Abdominis: A New Era—A Guide for Health and Fitness Professionals*. Peace River, Alberta: Munira Hudani PT Inc. p. 2.

179 Hudani, M. (2022). *Diastasis Rectus Abdominis: A New Era—A Guide for Health and Fitness Professionals*. Peace River, Alberta: Munira Hudani PT Inc. p. 4.

180 Hudani, M. (2022). *Diastasis Rectus Abdominis: A New Era—A Guide for Health and Fitness Professionals*. Peace River, Alberta: Munira Hudani PT Inc. p. 5.

181 Lee, D., & Hodges, P. W. (2016). Behavior of the linea alba during a curl-up task in diastasis rectus abdominis: An observational study. *Journal of Orthopaedic Sports and Physical Therapy*, *46*(7), 580–589.

182 Hudani, M. (2022). *Diastasis Rectus Abdominis: A New Era—A Guide for Health and Fitness Professionals*. Peace River, Alberta: Munira Hudani PT Inc. p. 5.

183 Hudani, M. (2022). *Diastasis Rectus Abdominis: A New Era—A Guide for Health and Fitness Professionals*. Peace River, Alberta: Munira Hudani PT Inc. p. 5.

184 Aljuraifani, R., Stafford, R. E., Hall, L. M., van den Hoorn, W., & Hodges, P. W. (2019). Task-specific differences in respiration-related activation of deep and superficial pelvic floor muscles. *Journal of Applied Physiology*, *126*(5), 1343–1351.

185 Smith, M. D., Coppieters, M. W., & Hodges, P. W. (2008). Is balance different in women with and without stress urinary incontinence? *Neurourology and Neurodynamics: Official Journal of the International Continence Society*, *27*, 71–78.

186 Sjödahl, J., Kvist, J., Gutke, A., & Öberg, B. (2009). The postural response of the pelvic floor muscles during limb movements: A methodological electromyography

study in parous women without lumbopelvic pain. *Clinical Biomechanics, 24*(2), 183-189.

187 Bordoni, B., & Zanier, E. (2013). Anatomical connections of the diaphragm: Influence of respiration on the body system. *Journal of Multidisciplinary Healthcare, 6,* 281-291.

188 Dugan, S. A., Lavender, M. D., Hebert-Beirne, J., & Brubaker, L. (2013). A pelvic floor fitness program for older women with urinary symptoms: A feasibility study. *American Journal of Physical Medicine and Rehabilitation, 5,* 672-676.

189 Foster, S. N., Spitznagle, T. M., Tuttle, L. J., Sutcliffe, S., et al. (2021). Hip and pelvic floor muscle strength in women with and without urgency and frequency—predominant lower urinary tract symptoms. *Journal of Women's Health Physical Therapy, 45*(3), 126-134.

190 Hodges, P. W., Sapsford, R., & Pengel, L. H. M. (2007). Postural and respiratory functions of the pelvic floor muscles. *Neurourology and Urodynamics: Official Journal of the International Continence Society, 26*(3), 362-371.

191 Talasz, H., Kremser, C., Kofler, M., Kalchschmid, E., Lechleitner, M., & Rudisch, A. (2011). Phase-locked parallel movement of diaphragm and pelvic floor during breathing and coughing—A dynamic MRI investigation in healthy females. *International Urogynecology Journal, 22*(1), 61-68.

192 Aljuraifani, R., Stafford, R. E., Hall, L. M., van den Hoorn, W., & Hodges, P. W. (2019). Task-specific differences in respiration-related activation of deep and superficial pelvic floor muscles. *Journal of Applied Physiology, 126*(5), 1343-1351.

193 Kaminoff, L. (2006). What yoga therapists should know about the anatomy of breathing. *International Journal of Yoga Therapy, 16*(1), 67-77.

194 Aliverti, A. et al. (1997). Cited by Celhay, I., Cordova, R., Miralles, R., Meza, F., et al. (2015). Effect of upper costal and costo-diaphragmatic breathing types on electromyographic activity of respiratory muscles. *Cranio, 33*(2), 100-106.

195 Green, M., & Moxham, J. (1985). The respiratory muscles. *Clinical Science, 68*(1), 1-10.

196 De Troyer, A., & Boriek, A. M. (2011). Mechanics of the respiratory muscles. *Comprehensive Physiology, 1*(3), 1273-1300.

197 Kaminoff, L. (2006). What yoga therapists should know about the anatomy of breathing. *International Journal of Yoga Therapy, 16*(1), 67-77.

198 Frank, C., Kobesova, A., & Kolar, P. (2013). Dynamic neuromuscular stabilization & sports rehabilitation. *International Journal of Sports Physical Therapy, 8*(1), 62-73.

199 Pickering, M., & Jones, J. F. (2002). The diaphragm: Two physiological muscles in one. *Journal of Anatomy, 201*(4), 305-312.

200 Pickering, M., & Jones, J. F. (2002). The diaphragm: Two physiological muscles in one. *Journal of Anatomy, 201*(4), 305-312.

201 Pickering, M., & Jones, J. F. (2002). The diaphragm: Two physiological muscles in one. *Journal of Anatomy, 201*(4), 305-312.

202 Kolář, P., Šulc, J., Kynčl, M., Šanda, J., et al. (2012). Postural function of the diaphragm in persons with and without chronic low back pain. *Journal of Orthopaedic and Sports Physical Therapy, 42*(4), 352-362.

203 Dres, M., & Demoule, A. (2020). Monitoring diaphragm function in the ICU. *Current Opinions in Critical Care, 26*(1), 18-25.

204 Hodges, P. W., Butler, J. E., McKenzie, D. K., & Gandevia, S. C. (1997). Contraction of the human diaphragm during rapid postural adjustments. *Journal of Physiology, 505*(2), 539-548.

205 Hodges, P. W., & Gandevia, S. C. (2000). Activation of the human diaphragm during a repetitive postural task. *Journal of Physiology, 522*(1), 165-175.

206 Hodges, P. W., & Gandevia, S. C. (2000). Changes in intra-abdominal pressure during postural and respiratory activation of the human diaphragm. *Journal of Applied Physiology, 89*(3), 967–976.

207 Nelson, N. (2012). Diaphragmatic breathing: The foundation of core stability. *Strength and Conditioning Journal, 34*(5), 34–40.

208 Kolar, P., Neuwirth, J., Sanda, J., Suchanek, V., et al. (2009). Analysis of diaphragm movement during tidal breathing and during its activation while breath holding using MRI synchronized with spirometry. *Physiological Research, 58*, 383–392.

209 Courtney, R. (2009). The functions of breathing and its dysfunctions and their relationship to breathing therapy. *International Journal of Osteopathic Medicine, 12*(3), 78–85.

210 O'Sullivan, P. B., & Beales, D. J. (2007). Changes in pelvic floor and diaphragm kinematics and respiratory patterns in subjects with sacroiliac joint pain following a motor learning intervention: A case series. *Manual Therapy, 12*(3), 209–218.

211 O'Sullivan, P. B., Beales, D. J., Beetham, J. A., Cripps, J., et al. (2002). Altered motor control strategies in subjects with sacroiliac joint pain during the active straight-leg-raise test. *Spine, 27*, E1–8.

212 McGill, S. M., Sharratt, M. T., & Seguin, J. P. (1995). Loads on spinal tissues during simultaneous lifting and ventilatory challenge. *Ergonomics, 38*, 1772–1792.

213 Akuthota, V., Ferreiro, A., Moore, T., & Fredericson, M. (2008). Core stability exercise principles. *Current Sports Medicine Reports, 7*(1), 39–44.

214 Sapsford, R. (2000). Explanation of medical terminology [letter]. *Neurourology and Urodynamics: Official Journal of the International Continence Society, 19*, 633.

215 Talasz, H., Kremser, C., Kofler, M., Kalchschmid, E., Lechleitner, M., & Rudisch, A. (2011). Phase-locked parallel movement of diaphragm and pelvic floor during breathing and coughing—A dynamic MRI investigation in healthy females. *International Urogynecology Journal, 22*(1), 61–68.

216 Key, J. (2013). "The core": Understanding it, and retraining its dysfunction. *Journal of Bodywork and Movement Therapies, 17*(4), 541–559.

217 Hodges, P. W., Gandevia, S. C., & Richardson, C. A. (1997). Contractions of specific abdominal muscles in postural tasks are effected by respiratory maneuvers. *Journal of Applied Physiology, 83*(3), 753–760.

218 Hodges, P. W., Gurfinkel, V. S., Brumagne, S., Smith, T. C., & Cordo, P. C. (2002). Coexistence of stability and mobility in postural control: Evidence from postural compensation for respiration. *Experimental Brain Research, 144*(3), 293–302.

219 Hodges, P. W., Kaigle Holm, A., Holm, S., Ekström, L., et al. (2003). Intervertebral stiffness of the spine is increased by evoked contraction of the transversus abdominis and the diaphragm: In vivo porcine studies. *Spine, 28*(23), 2594–2601.

220 Hodges, P. W., Sapsford, R., & Pengel, L. H. M. (2007). Postural and respiratory functions of the pelvic floor muscles. *Neurourology and Urodynamics: Official Journal of the International Continence Society, 26*(3), 362–371.

221 Hodges, P. W., & Gandevia, S. C. (2000). Activation of the human diaphragm during a repetitive postural task. *Journal of Physiology, 522*(1), 165–175.

222 Hodges, P. W., Kaigle Holm, A., Holm, S., Ekström, L., et al. (2003). Intervertebral stiffness of the spine is increased by evoked contraction of the transversus abdominis and the diaphragm: In vivo porcine studies. *Spine, 28*(23), 2594–2601.

223 Hodges, P. W., Gurfinkel, V. S., Brumagne, S., Smith, T. C., & Cordo, P. C. (2002). Coexistence of stability and mobility in postural control: Evidence from postural compensation for respiration. *Experimental Brain Research, 144*(3), 293–302.

224 Hodges, P. W., & Gandevia, S. C. (2000). Changes in intra-abdominal pressure during postural and respiratory activation of the human diaphragm. *Journal of Applied Physiology, 89*(3), 967–976.

225 Hodges, P. W., Heijnen, I., & Gandevia, S. C. (2001). Postural activity of the dia-phragm is reduced in humans when respiratory demand increases. *Journal of Physiology, 537*(Pt 3), 999–1008.

226 Hodges, P. W., Cresswell, A. G., Daggfeldt, K., & Thorstensson, A. (2001). In vivo measurement of the effect of intra-abdominal pressure on the human spine. *Journal of Biomechanics, 34*(3), 347–353.

227 Akuthota, V., Ferreiro, A., Moore, T., & Fredericson, M. (2008). Core stability exercise principles. *Current Sports Medicine Reports, 7*(1), 39–44.

228 Akuthota, V., & Nadler, S. F. (2004). Core strengthening. *Archives of Physical Med-icine and Rehabilitation, 85,* 86–92.

229 Richardson, C., Jull, G., Hodges, P., & Hides, J. (1999). *Therapeutic Exercise for Spinal Segmental Stabilization in Low Back Pain: Scientific Basis and Clinical Approach.* London: Churchill Livingstone.

230 Akuthota, V., Ferreiro, A., Moore, T., & Fredericson, M. (2008). Core stability exercise principles. *Current Sports Medicine Reports, 7*(1), 39–44.

231 Hodges, P. W. (1999). Is there a role for transversus abdominis in lumbo-pelvic stability? *Manual Therapy, 4*(2), 74–86.

232 Milanesi, R., & Caregnato, R. C. A. (2016). Intra-abdominal pressure: An integrative review. *Einstein (Sao Paulo), 14,* 423–430.

233 Cholewicki, J., Juluru, K., & McGill, S. M. (1999). Intra-abdominal pressure mech-anism for stabilizing the lumbar spine. *Journal of Biomechanics, 32*(1), 13–17.

234 Cholewicki, J., Ivancic, P. C., & Radebold, A. (2002). Can increased intra-abdominal pressure in humans be decoupled from trunk muscle co-contraction during steady state isometric exertions? *European Journal of Applied Physiology, 87*(2), 127–133.

235 Cholewicki, J., Ivancic, P. C., & Radebold, A. (2002). Can increased intra-abdominal pressure in humans be decoupled from trunk muscle co-contraction during steady state isometric exertions? *European Journal of Applied Physiology, 87*(2), 127–133.

236 Coulter, D. (2004). *Anatomy of Hatha Yoga: A Manual for Students, Teachers, and Practitioners.* Honesdale, PA: Body and Breath.

237 Cowan, P. T., Mudreac, A., & Varacallo, M. (2021). Anatomy, Back, Scapula. *StatPearls* [Internet]. Treasure Island, FL: StatPearls Publishing. Accessed on January 4, 2023 at https://pubmed.ncbi.nlm.nih.gov/30285370.

238 Long, R. (2011). Shoulder Kinematics in Yoga Part II: The Lower Trapezius and Ser-ratus Anterior. The Daily Bandha. Accessed on July 26, 2018 at www.dailybandha.com/2011/05/shoulder-kinematics-in-yoga-part-ii.html.

239 Hoppenfeld, S. (1976). *Physical Examination of the Spine and Extremities.* New York: Appleton-Century-Crofts. p. 30.

240 McQuade, K. J., Borstad, J., & de Oliveira, A. S. (2016). Critical and theoretical perspective on scapular stabilization: What does it really mean, and are we on the right track? *Physical Therapy, 96*(8), 1162–1169.

241 Nadler, S. F. (2004). Visual vignette: Injury in a throwing athlete: Understanding the kinetic chain. *American Journal of Physical Medical Rehabilitation, 83*(1), 79.

242 Kibler, W. B., & Livingston, B. P. (2001). Closed chain rehabilitation for upper and lower extremities. *Journal of American Academy of Orthopaedic Surgeons, 9,* 412–421.

243 Shinkle, J., Nesser, T. W., Demchak, T. J., & McManus, D. M. (2012). Effect of core strength on the measure of power in the extremities. *Journal of Strength and Con-ditioning Research, 26*(2), 373–380.

244 Stodden, D. F., Fleisig, G. S., McLean, S. P., & Andrews, J. R. (2005). Relationship of biomechanical factors to baseball pitching velocity: Within pitcher variation. *Journal of Applied Biomechanics, 21*(1), 44–56.

245 Hirashima, M., Kudo, K., & Ohtsuki, T. (2003). Utilization and compensation of interaction torques during ball throwing movements. *Journal of Neurophysiology, 89*(4), 1784–1796.

246 Marshall, R. N., & Elliott, B. C. (2000). Long axis rotation: The missing link in proximal to distal segmental sequencing. *Journal of Sports Science, 18,* 247–254.

247 Happee, R., & van der Helm, F. C. (1995). Control of shoulder muscles during goal-directed movements. *Journal of Biomechanics, 28,* 1170–1191.

248 Kibler, W. B., & McMullen, J. (2003). Rehabilitation of Scapular Dyskinesis. In S. B. Brotzman & K. E. Wilk (eds.) *Clinical Orthopedic Rehabilitation,* 2nd edition (pp. 244–250). St. Louis, MO: Mosby.

249 Hodges, P. W., & Richardson, C. A. (1997). Feedforward contraction of transversus abdominis is not influenced by direction of arm movement. *Experimental Brain Research, 114*(2), 362–370.

250 Kibler, W. B., Ludewig, P. M., McClure, P. W., Michener, L. A., Bak, K., & Sciascia, A. D. (2013). Clinical implications of scapular dyskinesis in shoulder injury: The 2013 consensus statement from the "Scapular Summit." *British Journal of Sports Medicine, 47*(14), 877–885.

251 Kibler, W. B., & McMullen, J. (2013). Rehabilitation of Scapular Dyskinesis. In S. B. Brotzman & K. E. Wilk (eds.) *Clinical Orthopedic Rehabilitation, 2nd edition* (pp. 244–250). St. Louis, MO: Mosby.

252 Seitz, A. L., McClure, P. W., Lynch, S. S., Ketchum, J. M., & Michener, L. A. (2012). Effects of scapular dyskinesis and scapular assistance test on subacromial space during static arm elevation. *Journal of Shoulder and Elbow Surgery, 21*(5), 631–640.

253 Baek, Y. J., Jung, Y. J., Son, J. I., Lim, O. B., & Yi, C. H. (2017). Comparison of muscle activity and trunk compensation during modified push-up plus exercises in individuals with scapular winging. *Isokinetics and Exercise Science, 25*(3), 201–207.

254 Hunter, D. J., Rivett, D. A., McKiernan, S., Smith, L., & Snodgrass, S. J. (2020). Relationship between shoulder impingement syndrome and thoracic posture. *Physical Therapy, 100*(4), 677–686.

255 Cortell-Tormo, J. M., García-Jaén, M., Chulvi-Medrano, I., Hernández-Sánchez, S., Lucas-Cuevas, Á. G., & Tortosa-Martínez, J. (2017). Influence of scapular position on the core musculature activation in the prone plank exercise. *Journal of Strength and Conditioning Research, 31*(8), 2255–2262.

256 Yach, B., & Linens, S. W. (2019). The relationship between breathing pattern disorders and scapular dyskinesis. *Athletic Training and Sports Health Care, 11*(2), 63–70.

257 Barrett, E., O'Keeffe, M., O'Sullivan, K., Lewis, J., & McCreesh, K. (2016). Is thoracic spine posture associated with shoulder pain, range of motion and function? A systematic review. *Manual Therapy, 26,* 38–46.

258 Lewis, J. S. (2011). Subacromial impingement syndrome: A musculoskeletal condition or a clinical illusion? *Physical Therapy Reviews, 16*(5), 388–398.

259 Park, S. W., Chen, Y. T., Thompson, L., Kjoenoe, A., et al. (2020). No relationship between the acromiohumeral distance and pain in adults with subacromial pain syndrome: A systematic review and meta-analysis. *Scientific Reports, 10*(1), 1–14.

260 Richards, K. V., Beales, D. J., Smith, A. L., O'Sullivan, P. B., & Straker, L. M. (2021). Is neck posture subgroup in late adolescence a risk factor for persistent neck pain in young adults? A prospective study. *Physical Therapy, 101*(3), pzab007.

261 Chester, R., Jerosch-Herold, C., Lewis, J., & Shepstone, L. (2018). Psychological factors are associated with the outcome of physiotherapy for people with shoulder pain: A multicentre longitudinal cohort study. *British Journal of Sports Medicine, 52*(4), 269–275.

262 Turgut, E., Duzgun, I., & Baltaci, G. (2017). Effects of scapular stabilization exercise training on scapular kinematics, disability, and pain in subacromial impingement:

A randomized controlled trial. *Archives of Physical Medicine and Rehabilitation*, 98(10), 1915–1923.

263 McQuade, K. J., Borstad, J., & de Oliveira, A. S. (2016). Critical and theoretical perspective on scapular stabilization: What does it really mean, and are we on the right track? *Physical Therapy*, 96(8), 1162–1169.

264 McQuade, K. J., Borstad, J., & de Oliveira, A. S. (2016). Critical and theoretical perspective on scapular stabilization: What does it really mean, and are we on the right track? *Physical Therapy*, 96(8), 1162–1169.

265 McQuade, K. J., Borstad, J., & de Oliveira, A. S. (2016). Critical and theoretical perspective on scapular stabilization: What does it really mean, and are we on the right track? *Physical Therapy*, 96(8), 1162–1169.

266 McQuade, K. J., Borstad, J., & de Oliveira, A. S. (2016). Critical and theoretical perspective on scapular stabilization: What does it really mean, and are we on the right track? *Physical Therapy*, 96(8), 1162–1169.

267 Nadler, S. F. (2004). Visual vignette: Injury in a throwing athlete: understanding the kinetic chain. *American Journal of Physical Medical Rehabilitation*, 83(1), 79.

268 Caldwell, C., Sahrmann, S., & Van Dillen, L. (2007). Use of a movement system impairment diagnosis for physical therapy in the management of a patient with shoulder pain. *Journal of Orthopaedic and Sports Physical Therapy*, 37(9), 551–563.

269 Glousman, R., Jobe, F., Tibone, J., Moynes, D., Antonelli, D., & Perry, J. (1988). Dynamic electromyographic analysis of the throwing shoulder with glenohumeral instability. *Journal of Bone and Joint Surgery. American Volume*, 70(2), 220–226.

270 Kibler, W. B., Ludewig, P. M., McClure, P. W., Michener, L. A., Bak, K., & Sciascia, A. D. (2013). Clinical implications of scapular dyskinesis in shoulder injury: The 2013 consensus statement from the "Scapular Summit." *British Journal of Sports Medicine*, 47(14), 877–885.

271 McMullen, J., & Uhl, T. L. (2000). A kinetic chain approach for shoulder rehabilitation. *Journal of Athletic Training*, 35(3), 329–337.

272 Scovazzo, M. L., Browne, A., Pink, M., Jobe, F. W., & Kerrigan, J. (1991). The painful shoulder during freestyle swimming: An electromyographic cinematographic analysis of twelve muscles. *American Journal of Sports Medicine*, 19(6), 577–582.

273 Seitz, A. L., McClure, P. W., Lynch, S. S., Ketchum, J. M., & Michener, L. A. (2012). Effects of scapular dyskinesis and scapular assistance test on subacromial space during static arm elevation. *Journal of Shoulder and Elbow Surgery*, 21(5), 631–640.

274 Seitz, A. L., McClure, P. W., Finucane, S., Boardman III, N. D., & Michener, L. A. (2011). Mechanisms of rotator cuff tendinopathy: Intrinsic, extrinsic, or both? *Clinical Biomechanics*, 26(1), 1–12.

275 Rice, S. G. (2003). Using the kinetic chain theory in clinical practice. *Current Sports Medicine Reports*, 2, 289–290.

276 Laudner, K. G., Wong, R., & Meister, K. (2019). The influence of lumbopelvic control on shoulder and elbow kinetics in elite baseball pitchers. *Journal of Shoulder and Elbow Surgery*, 28, 330–334.

277 Miyake, Y., Kobayashi, R., Kelepecz, D., & Nakajima, M. (2013). Core exercises elevate trunk stability to facilitate skilled motor behavior of the upper extremities. *Journal of Bodywork and Movement Therapies*, 17(2), 259–265.

278 Hazar, Z., Ulug, N., & Yuksel, I. (2014). Is there a relation between shoulder dysfunction and core instability? *Orthopaedic Journal of Sports Medicine*, 2(11_suppl3), 2325967114S00173.

279 Hazar, Z., Ulug, N., & Yuksel, I. (2014). Is there a relation between shoulder dysfunction and core instability? *Orthopaedic Journal of Sports Medicine*, 2(11_suppl3), 2325967114S00173.

280 Van de Velde, A., De Mey, K., Maenhout, A., Calders, P., & Cools, A. M. (2011). Scapular-muscle performance: Two training programs in adolescent swimmers. *Journal of Athletic Training, 46*(2), 160–167.

281 Merolla, G., De Santis, E., Sperling, J. W., Campi, F., Paladini, P., & Porcellini, G. (2010). Infraspinatus strength assessment before and after scapular muscles rehabilitation in professional volleyball players with scapular dyskinesis. *Journal of Shoulder and Elbow Surgery, 19*(8), 1256–1264.

282 Baek, Y. J., Jung, Y. J., Son, J. I., Lim, O. B., & Yi, C. H. (2017). Comparison of muscle activity and trunk compensation during modified push-up plus exercises in individuals with scapular winging. *Isokinetics and Exercise Science, 25*(3), 201–207.

283 Matsuo, K., & Palmer, J. B. (2008). Anatomy and physiology of feeding and swallowing: Normal and abnormal. *Physical Medicine and Rehabilitation Clinics of North America, 19*(4), 691–707.

284 Esling, J. (2006). States of the Glottis. In K. Brown (ed.) *Encyclopedia of Language and Linguistics*, pp. 129–132. Amsterdam: Elsevier. p. 129.

285 Massery, M. (2013, August 8). Glottal strategies—Massery PT—Mary Massery—If you can't breathe, you can't function [Video file]. Massery PT. Accessed on July 9, 2022 at www.youtube.com/watch?v=bF_uCPzYUDc.

286 Massery, M. (2013, August 8). Glottal strategies—Massery PT—Mary Massery—If you can't breathe, you can't function [Video file]. Massery PT. Accessed on July 9, 2022 at www.youtube.com/watch?v=bF_uCPzYUDc.

287 Talasz, H., Kofler, M., Kalchschmid, E., Pretterklieber, M., & Lechleitner, M. (2010). Breathing with the pelvic floor? Correlation of pelvic floor muscle function and expiratory flows in healthy young nulliparous women. *International Urogynecology Journal, 21*(4), 475–481.

288 Bordoni, B., & Zanier, E. (2013). Anatomic connections of the diaphragm: Influence of respiration on the body system. *Journal of Multidisciplinary Healthcare, 6*, 281–291.

289 Rudavsky, A., & Turner, T. (2020). Novel insight into the coordination between pelvic floor muscles and the glottis through ultrasound imaging: A pilot study. International *Urogynecology Journal, 31*(12), 2645–2652.

290 Massery, M. (2013, August 8). Glottal strategies—Massery PT—Mary Massery—If you can't breathe, you can't function [Video file]. Massery PT. Accessed on July 9, 2022 at www.youtube.com/watch?v=bF_uCPzYUDc.

291 Pelvic Guru (2019). Cervical, pelvic floor, and diaphragm connection: An interview with Susan Clinton. Accessed on March 6, 2022 at https://pelvicguru.com/cervical-pelvic-floor-and-diaphragm-connection-an-interview-with-susan-clinton.

292 Wiebe, J., & Clinton, S. (2022). From the Glottis to the Pelvic Floor: Making Clinical Connections. Julie Wiebe Physical Therapy, Inc. Accessed on June 15, 2022 at https://courses.juliewiebept.com/p/from-the-glottis-to-the-pelvic-floor-making-clinical-connections.

293 Herman & Wallace (2022). Breathing and the Diaphragm—Remote Course. Herman and Wallace Pelvic Rehabilitation Institute. Accessed on March 19, 2022 at https://hermanwallace.com/continuing-education-courses/breathing-and-the-diaphragm-remote-course.

294 Garner, G. (2019). Trauma Informed Yoga for Women's Health: The Voice Is Queen in the Pelvic Floor Kingdom. Embodia Inc. Accessed on February 12, 2019 at www.embodiaapp.com/webinars/38-trauma-informed-yoga-for-women-s-health-the-voice-is-queen-in-the-pelvic-floor-kingdom-dr-ginger-garner.

295 Bordoni, B. (2020). The five diaphragms in osteopathic manipulative medicine: Myofascial relationships, Part 1. *Cureus, 12*(4), e7794.

296 Bedekar, N. (2012). Pelvic floor muscle activation during singing: A pilot study. *Journal of the Association of Chartered Physiotherapists in Women's Health*, *110*, 27–32.
297 Taylor, M. (2011, September 13). The 3 Diaphragms Model [Video file]. DrMatthewJTaylor. Accessed on September 19, 2022 at www.youtube.com/watch?v=HTkFuPLZ3Uk.
298 Taylor, M. (2015, April 26). The 3 Diaphragms for Pain Relief [Video file]. DrMatthewJTaylor. Accessed on February 2, 2023 at www.youtube.com/watch?v=VbizoP44fys.
299 Kaminoff, L., & Matthews, A. (2012). *Yoga Anatomy*, 2nd edition. Champaign, IL: Human Kinetics.
300 Garcia-Falgueras, A. (2016). An introduction to proprioception concept in Pilates and yoga. *British Journal of Medicine and Medical Research*, *15*(3), 1–6.
301 Pilates, J. H., & Miller, W. J. (1945). *Return to Life through Contrology*. Cambridge, UK: Ravenio Books.
302 Lewit, K. (1980). Relation of faulty respiration to posture, with clinical implications. *Journal of the American Osteopathic Association*, *79*(8), 525–529.
303 Perri, M. A., & Halford, E. (2004). Pain and faulty breathing: A pilot study. *Journal of Bodywork and Movement Therapies*, *8*(4), 297–306.
304 Morris, C. E. (2015). The torsional upper crossed syndrome: A multi-planar update to Janda's model, with a case series introduction of the mid-pectoral fascial lesion as an associated etiological factor. *Journal of Bodywork and Movement Therapies*, *19*, 681–689.
305 Moore, M. K. (2004). Upper crossed syndrome and its relationship to cervicogenic headache. *Journal of Manipulative and Physiological Therapeutics*, *27*(6), 414–420.
306 Wallden, M. (2014). The middle-crossed syndrome—new insights into core function. *Journal of Bodywork and Movement Therapies*, *18*(4), 616–620.
307 Physiopedia (2022). Upper-Crossed Syndrome. Accessed on March 13, 2022 at www.physio-pedia.com/Upper-Crossed_Syndrome.
308 Physiopedia (2022). Upper-Crossed Syndrome. Accessed on March 13, 2022 at www.physio-pedia.com/Upper-Crossed_Syndrome.
309 Cuccia, A. M., Lottie, M., & Caradonna, D. (2008). Oral breathing and head posture. *Angel Orthodontist*, *78*(1), 77–82.
310 Koseki, T., Kakizaki, F., Hayashi, S., Nishida, N., & Itoh, M. (2019). Effect of forward head posture on thoracic shape and respiratory function. *Journal of Physical Therapy Science*, *31*(1), 63–68.
311 Kapreli, E., Vourazanis, E., & Strimpakos, N. (2008). Neck pain causes respiratory dysfunction. *Medical Hypotheses*, *70*(5), 1009–1013.
312 Zafar, H., Albarrati, A., Alghadir, A. H., & Iqbal, Z. A. (2018). Effects of different head-neck postures on the respiratory function in healthy males. *BioMedical Research International*. doi: 10.1155/2018/4518269.
313 Has, J., Park, Y., Kim, Y., Choi, Y., & Lyu, H. (2016). Effects of forward head posture on forced vital capacity and respiratory muscle activity. *Journal of Physical Therapy Science*, *28*(1), 128–131.
314 Physiopedia (2022). Lower-Crossed Syndrome. Accessed on March 13, 2022 at www.physio-pedia.com/Lower_Crossed_Syndrome.
315 Physiopedia (2022). Lower-Crossed Syndrome. Accessed on March 13, 2022 at www.physio-pedia.com/Lower_Crossed_Syndrome.
316 Physiopedia (2022). Lower-Crossed Syndrome. Accessed on March 13, 2022 at www.physio-pedia.com/Lower_Crossed_Syndrome.
317 Wallden, M. (2014). The middle crossed syndrome—new insights into core function. *Journal of Bodywork and Movement Therapies*, *18*(4), 616–620.
318 Key, J. (2013). "The core": Understanding it, and retraining its dysfunction. *Journal of Bodywork and Movement Therapies*, *17*(4), 541–559.

319 Key, J. (2010). The pelvic crossed syndromes: A reflection of imbalanced function in the myofascial envelope; a further exploration of Janda's work. *Journal of Bodywork and Movement Therapies, 14*(3), 299–301.

320 Key, J. (2013). "The core": Understanding it, and retraining its dysfunction. *Journal of Bodywork and Movement Therapies, 17*(4), 541–559.

321 Hodges, P. W., Cresswell, A. G., Daggfeldt, K., & Thorstensson, A. (2001). In vivo measurement of the effect of intra-abdominal pressure on the human spine. *Journal of Biomechanics, 34*(3), 347–353.

322 Cresswell, A. G., Blake, P. L., & Thorstensson, A. (1994). The effect of an abdominal muscle training program on intra-abdominal pressure. *Scandinavian Journal of Rehabilitation Medicine, 26*(2), 79–86.

323 Cresswell, A. G., Oddsson, L., & Thorstensson, A. (1994). The influence of sudden perturbations on trunk muscle activity and intra-abdominal pressure while standing. *Experimental Brain Research, 98,* 336–341.

324 Cresswell, A. G., Blake, P. L., & Thorstensson, A. (1994). The effect of an abdominal muscle training program on intra-abdominal pressure. *Scandinavian Journal of Rehabilitation Medicine, 26*(2), 79–86.

325 Talasz, H., Kremser, C., Kofler, M., Kalchschmid, E., Lechleitner, M., & Rudisch, A. (2011). Phase-locked parallel movement of diaphragm and pelvic floor during breathing and coughing—A dynamic MRI investigation in healthy females. *International Urogynecology Journal, 22*(1), 61–68.

326 Matsuo, K., & Palmer, J. B. (2008). Anatomy and physiology of feeding and swallowing: Normal and abnormal. *Physical Medicine and Rehabilitation Clinics of North America, 19*(4), 691–707.

327 Encyclopædia Britannica (2022). *Urination*. Accessed on March 16, 2022 at www.britannica.com/science/incontinence.

328 Whitehead, W. E., & Bharucha, A. E. (2010). Diagnosis and treatment of pelvic floor disorders: What's new and what to do. *Gastroenterology, 138*(4), 1231–1235.

329 Hosseini, S. M., & Jamshir, M. (2015). Valsalva maneuver and strain-related ECG changes. *Research in Cardiovascular Medicine, 4*(4), e28136.

330 Baessler, K., Metz, M., & Junginger, B. (2017). Valsalva versus straining: There is a distinct difference in resulting bladder neck and puborectalis muscle position. *Neurourology and Urodynamics: Official Journal of the International Continence Society, 36*(7), 1860–1866.

331 Baessler, K., Metz, M., & Junginger, B. (2017). Valsalva versus straining: There is a distinct difference in resulting bladder neck and puborectalis muscle position. *Neurourology and Urodynamics: Official Journal of the International Continence Society, 36*(7), 1860–1866.

332 Junginger, B., Vollhaber, H., & Baessler, K. (2018). Submaximal pelvic floor muscle contractions: Similar bladder-neck elevation, longer duration, less intra-abdominal pressure. *International Urogynecology Journal, 29*(11), 1681–1687.

333 Baessler, K., Metz, M., & Junginger, B. (2017). Valsalva versus straining: There is a distinct difference in resulting bladder neck and puborectalis muscle position. *Neurourology and Urodynamics: Official Journal of the International Continence Society, 36*(7), 1860–1866.

334 Rudavsky, A., & Turner, T. (2020). Novel insight into the coordination between pelvic floor muscles and the glottis through ultrasound imaging: A pilot study. *International Urogynecology Journal, 31*(12), 2645–2652.

335 Hosseini, S. M., & Jamshir, M. (2015). Valsalva maneuver and strain-related ECG changes. *Research in Cardiovascular Medicine, 4*(4), e28136.

336 Hosseini, S. M., & Jamshir, M. (2015). Valsalva maneuver and strain-related ECG changes. *Research in Cardiovascular Medicine, 4*(4), e28136.

337 Mens, J., van Dijke, G. H., Pool-Goudzwaard, A., van der Hulst, V., & Stam, H. (2006). Possible harmful effects of high intra-abdominal pressure on the pelvic girdle. *Journal of Biomechanics, 39*(4), 627–635.

338 Baessler, K., Metz, M., & Junginger, B. (2017). Valsalva versus straining: There is a distinct difference in resulting bladder neck and puborectalis muscle position. *Neurourology and Urodynamics: Official Journal of the International Continence Society, 36*(7), 1860–1866.

339 Junginger, B., Vollhaber, H., & Baessler, K. (2018). Submaximal pelvic floor muscle contractions: Similar bladder-neck elevation, longer duration, less intra-abdominal pressure. *International Urogynecology Journal, 29*(11), 1681–1687.

340 Hodges, P. W., & Gandevia, S. C. (2000). Changes in intra-abdominal pressure during postural and respiratory activation of the human diaphragm. *Journal of Applied Physiology, 89*(3), 967–976.

341 Hodges, P. W., Gurfinkel, V. S., Brumagne, S., Smith, T. C., & Cordo, P. C. (2002). Coexistence of stability and mobility in postural control: Evidence from postural compensation for respiration. *Experimental Brain Research, 144*(3), 293–302.

342 Hodges, P. W., Heijnen, I., & Gandevia, S. C. (2001). Postural activity of the diaphragm is reduced in humans when respiratory demand increases. *Journal of Physiology, 537*(Pt 3), 999–1008.

343 Hodges, P. W., Cresswell, A. G., Daggfeldt, K., & Thorstensson, A. (2001). In vivo measurement of the effect of intra-abdominal pressure on the human spine. *Journal of Biomechanics, 34*(3), 347–353.

344 Cholewicki, J., Juluru, K., & McGill, S. M. (1999). Intra-abdominal pressure mechanism for stabilizing the lumbar spine. *Journal of Biomechanics, 32*(1), 13–17.

345 Cobb, W. S., Burns, J. M., Kercher, K. W., Matthews, B. D., Norton, H. J., & Heniford, B. T. (2005). Normal intraabdominal pressure in healthy adults. *Journal of Surgical Research, 129*(2), 231–235.

346 Cobb, W. S., Burns, J. M., Kercher, K. W., Matthews, B. D., Norton, H. J., & Heniford, B. T. (2005). Normal intraabdominal pressure in healthy adults. *Journal of Surgical Research, 129*(2), 231–235.

347 Frank, C., Kobesova, A., & Kolar, P. (2013). Dynamic neuromuscular stabilization and sports rehabilitation. *International Journal of Sports Physical Therapy, 8*(1), 62–73.

348 Leahey, P. M. (1999). Active Release Techniques: A Logical Approach to Soft Tissue Treatment. In W. J. Hammer (ed.) *Functional Soft Tissue Examination and Treatment by Manual Methods*, 2nd edition, pp. 549–552. Gaithersburg, MD: Aspen.

349 Spina, A. A. (2007). External coxa saltans (snapping hip) treated with Active Release Techniques: A case report. *Journal of the Canadian Chiropractic Association, 51*(1), 23–29.

350 Massery, M. (2006). Multisystem Consequences of Impaired Breathing Mechanics and/or Postural Control. In D. Frownfelter & E. Dean (eds.) *Cardiovascular and Pulmonary Physical Therapy Evidence and Practice*, 4th edition, pp. 695–717. St. Louis, MO: Elsevier Health Sciences. p. 706.

Chapter 6

1 Bradley, H., & Esformes, J. D. (2014). Breathing pattern disorders and functional movement. *International Journal of Sports Physical Therapy, 9*(1), 28–39.

2 Streeter, C. C., Gerbarg, P. L., Saper, R. B., Ciraulo, D. A., & Brown, R. P. (2012). Effects of yoga on the autonomic nervous system, gamma-aminobutyric-acid, and allostasis in epilepsy, depression, and post-traumatic stress disorder. *Medical Hypotheses, 78*(5), 571–579.

3   Danucalov, M. A. D., Simoes, R. S., Kozasa, E. H., & Leite, J. R. (2008). Cardiore-spiratory and metabolic changes during yoga sessions: The effects of respiratory exercises and meditation practices. *Applied Psychophysiology and Biofeedback, 33*(2), 77–81.

4   Green, M., & Moxham, J. (1985). The respiratory muscles. *Clinical Science, 68*(1), 1–10.

5   Kaminoff, L. (2006). What yoga therapists should know about the anatomy of breathing. *International Journal of Yoga Therapy, 16*(1), 67–77.

6   Coulter, D. (2004). *Anatomy of Hatha Yoga: A Manual for Students, Teachers, and Practitioners.* Honesdale, PA: Body and Breath. p. 74.

7   Lofrese, J. J., Tupper, C., Denault, D., & Lappin, S. L. (2022). Physiology, Residual Volume. *StatPearls.* Treasure Island, FL: StatPearls Publishing. Accessed on July 12, 2022 at www.ncbi.nlm.nih.gov/books/NBK493170.

8   Chapman, E. B., Hansen-Honeycutt, J., Nasypany, A., Baker, R. T., & May, J. (2016). A clinical guide to the assessment and treatment of breathing pattern disorders in the physically active: Part 1. *International Journal of Sports Physical Therapy, 11*(5), 803–809.

9   Coulter, D. (2004). *Anatomy of Hatha Yoga: A Manual for Students, Teachers, and Practitioners.* Honesdale, PA: Body and Breath. p. 74.

10 Chapman, E. B., Hansen-Honeycutt, J., Nasypany, A., Baker, R. T., & May, J. (2016). A clinical guide to the assessment and treatment of breathing pattern disorders in the physically active: Part 1. *International Journal of Sports Physical Therapy, 11*(5), 803–809.

11 Perri, M. A., & Halford, E. (2004). Pain and faulty breathing: A pilot study. *Journal of Bodywork and Movement Therapies, 8*(4), 297–306.

12 De Troyer, A., & Estenne, M. (1984). Cited in Perri, M. A., & Halford, E. (2004). Pain and faulty breathing: A pilot study. *Journal of Bodywork and Movement Therapies, 8*(4), 297–306.

13 De Troyer, A., & Boriek, A. M. (2011) Mechanics of the respiratory muscles. *Comprehensive Physiology, 1,* 1273–1300.

14 Key, J. (2013). "The core": Understanding it, and retraining its dysfunction. *Journal of Bodywork and Movement Therapies, 17*(4), 541–559.

15 Kolář, P., Šulc, J., Kynčl, M., Šanda, J., et al. (2012) and Kolar, P., Kobesova, A., Valouchova, P., & Bitnar, P. (2014) cited in Chapman, E. B., Hansen-Honeycutt, J., Nasypany, A., Baker, R. T., & May, J. (2016). A clinical guide to the assessment and treatment of breathing pattern disorders in the physically active: Part 1. *International Journal of Sports Physical Therapy, 11*(5), 803–809.

16 Chapman, E. B., Hansen-Honeycutt, J., Nasypany, A., Baker, R. T., & May, J. (2016). A clinical guide to the assessment and treatment of breathing pattern disorders in the physically active: Part 1. *International Journal of Sports Physical Therapy, 11*(5), 803–809.

17 Massery, M. (2006). Multisystem Consequences of Impaired Breathing Mechanics and/or Postural Control. In D. Frownfelter & E. Dean (eds.) *Cardiovascular and Pulmonary Physical Therapy Evidence and Practice,* 4th edition, pp. 695–717. St. Louis, MO: Elsevier Health Sciences. p. 695.

18 Kaminoff, L. (2006). What yoga therapists should know about the anatomy of breathing. *International Journal of Yoga Therapy, 16*(1), 67–77.

19 Leistad, R. B., Sand, T., Westgaard, R. H., Nilsen, K. B., & Stovner, L. J. (2006). Stress-induced pain and muscle activity in patients with migraine and tension-type headache. *Cephalalgia, 26*(1), 64–73.

20 Huska (1997), quoted in Perri, M. A., & Halford, E. (2004). Pain and faulty breathing: A pilot study. *Journal of Bodywork and Movement Therapies, 8*(4), 297–306.

21 Chapman, E. B., Hansen-Honeycutt, J., Nasypany, A., Baker, R. T., & May, J. (2016). A clinical guide to the assessment and treatment of breathing pattern disorders in the physically active: Part 1. *International Journal of Sports Physical Therapy, 11*(5), 803–809.

22 Gray's 1995 quoted in Perri, M. A., & Halford, E. (2004). Pain and faulty breathing: A pilot study. *Journal of Bodywork and Movement Therapies, 8*(4), 297–306.

23 Huska (1997), quoted in Perri, M. A., & Halford, E. (2004). Pain and faulty breathing: A pilot study. *Journal of Bodywork and Movement Therapies, 8*(4), 297–306.

24 Chapman, E. B., Hansen-Honeycutt, J., Nasypany, A., Baker, R. T., & May, J. (2016). A clinical guide to the assessment and treatment of breathing pattern disorders in the physically active: Part 1. *International Journal of Sports Physical Therapy, 11*(5), 803–809.

25 Page, P. (2011). Cervicogenic headaches: An evidence-led approach to clinical management. *International Journal of Sports Physical Therapy, 6*(3), 254–266.

26 Massery, M. (2006). Multisystem Consequences of Impaired Breathing Mechanics and/or Postural Control. In D. Frownfelter & E. Dean (eds.) *Cardiovascular and Pulmonary Physical Therapy Evidence and Practice*, 4th edition, pp. 695–717. St. Louis, MO: Elsevier Health Sciences. p. 706.

27 Jansens, L., Brumagne, S., Polspoel, K., Troosters, T., & McConnell, A. (2010). The effect of inspiratory muscles fatigue on postural control in people with and without recurrent low back pain. *Spine, 35*(10), 1088–1094.

28 Perri, M. A., & Halford, E. (2004). Pain and faulty breathing: A pilot study. *Journal of Bodywork and Movement Therapies, 8*(4), 297–306.

29 Okuro, R. T., Morcillo, A. M., Ribeiro, M. A., Sakano, E., Conti, P. B., & Ribeiro, J. D. (2011). Mouth breathing and forward head posture: Effects on respiratory biomechanics and exercise capacity in children. *Jornal Brasileiro de Pneumologia, 37*(4), 471–479.

30 Brilla, L. R., & Kauffman, T. H. (2014). Effect of inspiratory muscle training and core exercise training on core functional tests. *Journal of Exercise Physiology Online, 17*(3), 12–20.

31 Segizbaeva, M. O., Timofeev, N. N., Donina, Z. A., Kur'yanovich, E. N., & Aleksandrova, N. P. (2015). Effects of inspiratory muscle training on resistance to fatigue of respiratory muscles during exhaustive exercise. *Advances in Experimental Medicine and Biology, 840*, 35–43.

32 Chatham, K., Baldwin, J., Griffiths, H., Summers, L., & Enright, S. (1999). Inspiratory muscle training improves shuttle run performance in healthy subjects. *Physiotherapy, 85*(12), 676–683.

33 Tong, T. K., McConnell, A. K., Lin, H., Nie, J., Zhang, H., & Wang, J. (2016). "Functional" inspiratory and core muscle training enhances running performance and economy. *Journal of Strength and Conditioning Research, 30*(10), 2942–2951.

34 De Troyer, A., & Boriek, A. M. (2011). Mechanics of the respiratory muscles. *Comprehensive Physiology, 1*, 1273–1300.

35 Hodges, P., & Gandevia, S. (2000). Changes in intra-abdominal pressure during postural and respiratory lactivation of the human diaphragm. *Journal of Applied Physiology, 89*, 967–976.

36 De Troyer, A., & Boriek, A. M. (2011) Mechanics of the respiratory muscles. *Comprehensive Physiology, 1*, 1273–1300.

37 Neumann, P., & Gill, V. (2002). Pelvic floor and abdominal muscle interaction: EMG activity and intra-abdominal pressure. *International Urogynecology Journal, 13*(2), 125–132.

38 Tirkes, T., Sandrasegaran, K., Patel, A. A., Hollar, M. A., et al. (2012). Peritoneal and retroperitoneal anatomy and its relevance for cross-sectional imaging. *Radiographics, 32*(2), 437–451.

39 Koch, L. (2012). *The Psoas Book.* Felton, CA: Guinea Pig Publishing. p. 42.

40 Littlejohn, C. (2010, June). The Psoas: Release or Resolve? Accessed on January 4, 2023 at https://thaihealingalliance.com/wp-content/uploads/The_Psoas_Release_or_Resolve_-_Carmen_Littlejohn.pdf.

41 Levine, P. A. (1997). *Waking the Tiger: Healing Trauma—The Innate Capacity to Transform Overwhelming Experiences.* Berkeley, CA: North Atlantic Books.

42 Koch, L. (2012). *Core Awareness: Enhancing Yoga, Pilates, Exercise, and Dance,* revised edition. Berkeley, CA: North Atlantic Books.

43 Long, R. (2007). Scientific Keys. Activating Your Accessories: The Accessory Muscles of Breath—Part II. Bandha Yoga, Inc. Accessed on August 17, 2018 at www.bandhayoga.com/keys_access2.html.

44 Santaguida, P. L., & McGill, S. M. (1995). The psoas major muscle: A three-dimensional geometric study. *Journal of Biomechanics, 28*(3), 343–345.

45 Herold, A. (2015). Neurogenic tremor through TRE tension, stress and trauma releasing exercises according to D. Berceli in the treatment of post-traumatic stress disorder (PTSD). *Psychological Counseling and Psychotherapy, 2*(1–2), 76–84.

46 CliftonSmith, T., & Rowley, J. (2011). Breathing pattern disorders and physiotherapy: Inspiration for our profession. *Physical Therapy Review, 16,* 75–86.

47 Physiopedia (2022). Breathing Pattern Disorders. Accessed on January 4, 2023 at www.physio-pedia.com/Breathing_Pattern_Disorders.

48 Kaminoff, L. (2006). What yoga therapists should know about the anatomy of breathing. *International Journal of Yoga Therapy, 16*(1), 67–77.

49 Perri, M. A., & Halford, E. (2004). Pain and faulty breathing: A pilot study. *Journal of Bodywork and Movement Therapies, 8*(4), 297–306.

50 National Center for Biotechnology Information (2022). Paradoxical respiration. National Library of Medicine. Accessed on April 29, 2022 at www.ncbi.nlm.nih.gov/medgen/534076.

51 Lewitt, K. (1980). Relationship of faulty respiration to posture, with clinical implications. *Journal of the American Osteopath Association, 79*(8), 525–528.

52 Yach, B., & Linens, S. W. (2019). The relationship between breathing pattern disorders and scapular dyskinesis. *Athletic Training and Sports Health Care, 11*(2), 63–70.

53 Roussel, N. A., Nijs, J., & Truijen, S. (2007). Low back pain: Climetric properties of the Tredelenburg test, active straight leg raise test and breathing pattern during active straight leg raising. *Journal of Manipulative Physiological Therapy, 30*(4), 270–278.

54 Smith, M., Russell, A., & Hodges, P. (2006). Disorders of breathing and continence have a stronger association with back pain than obesity and physical activity. *Australian Journal of Physiotherapy, 52,* 11–16.

55 Kapreli, E., Vourazanis, E., Billis, E., Oldham, J. A., & Strimpakos, N. (2009). Respiratory dysfunction in chronic neck pain patients: A pilot study. *Cephalalgia, 29*(7), 701–710.

56 Perri, M. A., & Halford, E. (2004). Pain and faulty breathing: A pilot study. *Journal of Bodywork and Movement Therapy, 8,* 297–306.

57 Hruska, R. (1997). Influences of dysfunctional respiratory mechanics on orofacial pain. *Dental Clinics of North America, 41*(2), 211–227.

58 Bradley, H., & Esformes, J. D. (2014). Breathing pattern disorders and functional movement. *International Journal of Sports Physical Therapy, 9*(1), 28–39.

59   Celhay, I., Cordova, R., Miralles, R., Meza, F., et al. (2015). Effect of upper costal and costo-diaphragmatic breathing types on electromyographic activity of respiratory muscles. *Cranio, 33*(2), 100–106.

60   Cavenaugh, B. (2021). End-of-Life Signs. Beth Cavenaugh. Accessed on January 5, 2022 at www.bethcavenaugh.com/blog/end-of-life-signs-how-to-tell-when-a-hospice-patient-is-close-to-the-moment-of-death.

61   Hansen-Honeycutt, J., Chapman, E. B., Nasypany, A., Baker, R. T., & May, J. (2016). A clinical guide to the assessment and treatment of breathing pattern disorders in the physically active: Part 2, A case series. *International Journal of Sports Physical Therapy, 11*(6), 971–979.

62   Sakellari, V., Bronstein, A. M., Corna, S., Hammon, C. A., Jones, S., & Wolsley, C. J. (1997). The effects of hyperventilation on postural control mechanisms. *Brain: A Journal of Neurology, 120*(9), 1659–1673.

63   Jansens, L., Brumagne, S., Polspoel, K., Troosters, T., & McConnell, A. (2010). The effect of inspiratory muscles fatigue on postural control in people with and without recurrent low back pain. *Spine, 35*(10), 1088–1094.

64   Chapman, E. B., Hansen-Honeycutt, J., Nasypany, A., Baker, R. T., & May, J. (2016). A clinical guide to the assessment and treatment of breathing pattern disorders in the physically active: Part 1. *International Journal of Sports Physical Therapy, 11*(5), 803–809.

65   Anderson, B. E., & Bliven, K. C. H. (2017). The use of breathing exercises in the treatment of chronic, nonspecific low back pain. *Journal of Sport Rehabilitation, 26*(5), 452–458.

66   Roussel, N., Nijs, J., Truijen, S., Vervecken, L., Mottram, S., & Stassijns, G. (2009). Altered breathing patterns during lumbopelvic motor control tests in chronic low back pain: A case-control study. *European Spine Journal, 18*(7), 1066–1073.

67   Diatchencko, L., Nackley, A., Slade, G. D., Fillingim, R. B., & Maixner, W. (2006). Idiopathic pain disorders: Pathways of vulnerability. *Pain, 123*(3), 226–230.

68   Han, J. N., Stegen, K., De Valck, C., Clement, J., & Van de Woestijne, K. P. (1996). Influence of breathing therapy on complaints, anxiety and breathing pattern in patients with hyperventilation syndrome and anxiety disorders. *Journal of Psychosomatic Research, 41*(5), 481–493.

69   Janssens, L., Brumagne, S., Polspoel, K., Troosters, T., & McConnell, A. (2010). The effect of inspiratory muscles fatigue on postural control in people with and without recurrent low back pain. *Spine, 35*(10), 1088–1094.

70   O'Sullivan, P. B., & Beales, D. J. (2007). Changes in pelvic floor and diaphragm kinematics and respiratory patterns in subjects with sacroiliac joint pain following a motor learning intervention: A case series. *Manual Therapy, 12*(3), 209–218.

71   CliftonSmith, T., & Rowley, J. (2011). Breathing pattern disorders and physiotherapy: Inspiration for our profession. *Physical Therapy Reviews, 16*(1), 75–86.

72   Kolář, P., Šulc, J., Kynčl, M., Šanda, J., et al. (2012). Postural function of the diaphragm in persons with and without chronic low back pain. *Journal of Orthopaedic and Sports Physical Therapy, 42*(4), 352–362.

73   Hodges, P. W., & Moseley, G. L. (2003). Pain and motor control of the lumbopelvic region: Effect and possible mechanisms. *Journal of Electromyography and Kinesiology, 13*(4), 361–370.

74   Bradley, H., & Esformes, J. D. (2014). Breathing pattern disorders and functional movement. *International Journal of Sports Physical Therapy, 9*(1), 28–39.

75   Nestor, J. (2020). *Breath: The New Science of a Lost Art.* New York: Penguin.

76   Yi, L. C., Jardim, J. R., Inoue, D. P., & Pignatari, S. S. (2008). The relationship between excursion of the diaphragm and curvatures of the spinal column in mouth breathing children. *Journal of Pediatrics, 84*(2), 171–177.

77 Cuccia, A. M., Lottie, M., & Caradonna, D. (2008). Oral breathing and head posture. *Angel Orthodontics*, *78*(1), 77–82.

78 Neiva, P. D., Kirkwood, R. N., & Godinho, R. (2009). Orientation and position of head posture, scapula and thoracic spine in mouth-breathing children. *International Journal of Pediatric Otorhinolaryngology*, *73*(2), 227–236.

79 Okuro, R. T., Morcillo, A. M., Ribeiro, M. A., Sakano, E., Conti, P. B., & Ribeiro, J. D. (2011). Mouth breathing and forward head posture: Effects on respiratory biomechanics and exercise capacity in children. *Jornal Brasileiro de Pneumologia*, *37*(4), 471–479.

80 Huggare, J. A., & Laine-Alava, M. T. (1997). Nasorespiratory function and head posture. *American Journal of Orthodontics and Dentofacial Orthopedics*, *112*(5), 507–511.

81 Zafar, H., Albarrati, A., Alghadir, A. H., & Iqbal, Z. A. (2018). Effects of different head-neck postures on the respiratory function in healthy males. *BioMedical Research International*. doi: 10.1155/2018/4518269.

82 Lima, L. C., Barauna, M. A., Sologurem, M. J., Canto, R. S., & Gastaldi, A. C. (2004). Postural alterations in children with mouth breathing assessed by computerized biophotogrammetry. *Journal of Applied Oral Science*, *12*(3), 232–237.

83 Correa, E. C., & Berin, F. (2008). Mouth breathing syndrome: Cervical muscles recruitment during nasal inspiration before and after respiratory and postural exercises on Swiss ball. *International Journal of Pediatric Otorhinolaryngology*, *72*(9), 1335–1343.

84 Okuro, R. T., Morcillo, A. M., Ribeiro, M. A., Sakano, E., Conti, P. B., & Ribeiro, J. D. (2011). Mouth breathing and forward head posture: Effects on respiratory biomechanics and exercise capacity in children. *Jornal Brasileiro de Pneumologia*, *37*(4), 471–479.

85 Bachour, A., & Maasilta, P. (2004). Mouth breathing compromises adherence to nasal continuous positive airway pressure therapy. *Chest*, *126*(4), 1248–1254.

86 Mayo Clinic (2022). Sleep apnea. Accessed on April 30, 2022 at www.mayoclinic.org/diseases-conditions/sleep-apnea/symptoms-causes/syc-20377631.

87 American Academy of Sleep Medicine (2014, July 29). Rising prevalence of sleep apnea in US threatens public. Accessed on April 30, 2022 at https://aasm.org/rising-prevalence-of-sleep-apnea-in-u-s-threatens-public-health.

88 Erturk, N., Calik-Kutukcu, E., Arikan, H., Savci, S., et al. (2020). The effectiveness of oropharyngeal exercises compared to inspiratory muscle training in obstructive sleep apnea: A randomized controlled trial. *Heart and Lung*, *49*(6), 940–948.

89 Erturk, N., Calik-Kutukcu, E., Arikan, H., Savci, S., et al. (2020). The effectiveness of oropharyngeal exercises compared to inspiratory muscle training in obstructive sleep apnea: A randomized controlled trial. *Heart and Lung*, *49*(6), 940–948.

90 Segizbaeva, M. O., Timofeev, N. N., Donina, Z. A., Kur'yanovich, E. N., & Aleksandrova, N. P. (2015). Effects of inspiratory muscle training on resistance to fatigue of respiratory muscles during exhaustive exercise. *Advances in Experimental Medicine and Biology*, *840*, 35–43.

91 Brilla, L. R., & Kauffman, T. H. (2014). Effect of inspiratory muscle training and core exercise training on core functional tests. *Journal of Exercise Physiology Online*, *17*(3), 12–20.

92 Chatham, K., Baldwin, J., Griffiths, H., Summers, L., & Enright, S. (1999). Inspiratory muscle training improves shuttle run performance in healthy subjects. *Physiotherapy*, *85*(12), 676–683.

93 Shei, R. J. (2020). Training load influences the response to inspiratory muscle training. *Journal of Sports Science and Medicine*, *19*(4), 772–773.

94 Tong, T. K., McConnell, A. K., Lin, H., Nie, J., Zhang, H., & Wang, J. (2016). "Functional" inspiratory and core muscle training enhances running performance and economy. *Journal of Strength and Conditioning Research, 30*(10), 2942–2951.

95 Nobre e Souza, M. A., Lima, M. J. V., Martins, G. B., Nobre, R. A., et al. (2013). Inspiratory muscle training improves antireflux barrier in GERD patients. *American Journal of Physiology-Gastrointestinal and Liver Physiology, 305*(11), G862–G867.

96 Liu, X. C., Pan, L., Hu, Q., Dong, W. P., Yan, J. H., & Dong, L. (2014). Effects of yoga training in patients with chronic obstructive pulmonary disease: A systematic review and meta-analysis. *Journal of Thoracic Disease, 6*(6), 795–802.

97 Giacomini, M. B., da Silva, A. M. V., Weber, L. M., & Monteiro, M. B. (2016). The Pilates method increases respiratory muscle strength and performance as well as abdominal muscle thickness. *Journal of Bodywork and Movement Therapies, 20*(2), 258–264.

98 DeLuca, N. D., Vajta Gomez, J. P., Vital, I., Cahalin, L. P., & Campos, M. A. (2020). The impact of yoga on inspiratory muscle performance in veterans with COPD: A pilot study. *International Journal of Yoga Therapy, 31*(1), Article_4.

99 Yelvar, G. D. Y., Çirak, Y., Demir, Y. P., Dalkilinç, M., & Bozkurt, B. (2016). Immediate effect of manual therapy on respiratory functions and inspiratory muscle strength in patients with COPD. *International Journal of Chronic Obstructive Pulmonary Disease, 11*, 1353–1357.

100 Cruz-Montecinos, C., Godoy-Olave, D., Contreras-Briceño, F. A., Gutiérrez, P., et al. (2017). The immediate effect of soft tissue manual therapy intervention on lung function in severe chronic obstructive pulmonary disease. *International Journal of Chronic Obstructive Pulmonary Disease, 12*, 691–696.

101 Prosko, S. (2019). Breathing and Pranayama in Pain Care. In N. Pearson, S. Prosko, & M. Sullivan (eds.) *Yoga and Science in Pain Care: Treating the Person in Pain* (pp. 141–157). London: Singing Dragon. p. 151.

102 Jafari et al. (2017), quoted in Prosko, S. (2019). Breathing and Pranayama in Pain Care. In N. Pearson, S. Prosko, & M. Sullivan (eds.) *Yoga and Science in Pain Care: Treating the Person in Pain* (pp. 141–157). London: Singing Dragon. p. 151.

103 Coulter, D. (2004). *Anatomy of Hatha Yoga: A Manual for Students, Teachers, and Practitioners.* Honesdale, PA: Body and Breath. p. 105.

104 Long, R. (2007). Scientific Keys. Activating Your Accessories: The Accessory Muscles of Breath—Part I. Bandha Yoga, Inc. Accessed on February 10, 2023 at www.bandhayoga.com/keys_access.html.

105 De Mayo, T., Miralles, R., Barrero, D., Bulboa, A., et al. (2005). Breathing type and body position effects on sternocleidomastoid and suprahyoid EMG activity. *Journal of Oral Rehabilitation, 32*(7), 487–494.

106 Celhay, I., Cordova, R., Miralles, R., Meza, F., et al. (2015). Effect of upper costal and costo-diaphragmatic breathing types on electromyographic activity of respiratory muscles. *Cranio, 33*(2), 100–106.

107 De Mayo, T., Miralles, R., Barrero, D., Bulboa, A., et al. (2005). Breathing type and body position effects on sternocleidomastoid and suprahyoid EMG activity. *Journal of Oral Rehabilitation, 32*(7), 487–494.

108 Haugstad, G. K., Haugstad, T. S., Kirste, U. M., Leganger, S., et al. (2006). Posture, movement patterns, and body awareness in women with chronic pelvic pain. *Journal of Psychosomatic Research, 61*(5), 637–644.

109 Lundberg, U., Dohns, I. E., Melin, B., & Sandsjö, L. (1999). Psychophysiological stress responses, muscle tension, and neck and shoulder pain among supermarket cashiers. *Journal of Occupational Health Psychology, 4*(3), 245–255.

110 Helou, L. B., Rosen, C. A., Wang, W., & Abbott, K. V. (2018). Intrinsic laryngeal muscle response to a public speech preparation stressor. *Journal of Speech, Language, and Hearing Research, 61*(7), 1525–1543.

111 Massery, M. (2006). Multisystem Consequences of Impaired Breathing Mechanics and/or Postural Control. In D. Frownfelter & E. Dean (eds.) *Cardiovascular and Pulmonary Physical Therapy Evidence and Practice*, 4th edition, pp. 695–717. St. Louis, MO: Elsevier Health Sciences. p. 706.

112 Sukel, K. (2019, August 25). Neuroanatomy: The Basics. Dana Foundation. Accessed on March 31, 2022 at https://dana.org/article/neuroanatomy-the-basics.

113 Rachel, N. (2020). The Autonomic Nervous System Explained. Natalia Rachel. Accessed on March 31, 2022 at www.nataliarachel.com/articles-general/the-autonomic-nervous-system-explained.

114 Taylor, M. (2011, September 13). The 3 Diaphragms Model [Video file]. DrMatthewJTaylor. Accessed on September 19, 2022 at www.youtube.com/watch?v=HTkFuPLZ3Uk.

115 Perri, M. A., & Halford, E. (2004). Pain and faulty breathing: A pilot study. *Journal of Bodywork and Movement Therapies, 8*(4), 297–306.

116 Kobuch, S., Fazalbhoy, A., Brown, R., Macefield, V. G., & Henderson, L. A. (2018). Muscle sympathetic nerve activity-coupled changes in brain activity during sustained muscle pain. *Brain and Behavior, 8*(3), 1–12.

117 McManus, C. (2012). Stress-induced hyperalgesia: Clinical implications for the physical therapist. *Orthopedic Physical Therapy Practice, 24*(3), 165–168.

118 Kobuch, S., Fazalbhoy, A., Brown, R., Macefield, V. G., & Henderson, L. A. (2018). Muscle sympathetic nerve activity-coupled changes in brain activity during sustained muscle pain. *Brain and Behavior, 8*(3), e00888.

119 Jewson, J. L., Lambert, E. A., Docking, S., Storr, M., Lambert, G. W., & Gaida, J. E. (2017). Pain duration is associated with increased muscle sympathetic nerve activity in patients with Achilles tendinopathy. *Scandinavian Journal of Medicine and Science in Sports, 27*(12), 1942–1949.

120 Smith, M. D., Russell, A., & Hodges, P. W. (2006). Disorders of breathing and continence have a stronger association with back pain than obesity and physical activity. *Australian Journal of Physiotherapy, 52*(1), 11–16.

121 Perri, M. A., & Halford, E. (2004). Pain and faulty breathing: A pilot study. *Journal of Bodywork and Movement Therapies, 8*(4), 297–306.

122 Perri, M. A., & Halford, E. (2004). Pain and faulty breathing: A pilot study. *Journal of Bodywork and Movement Therapies, 8*(4), 297–306.

123 Perri, M. A., & Halford, E. (2004). Pain and faulty breathing: A pilot study. *Journal of Bodywork and Movement Therapies, 8*(4), 297–306.

124 Diamond, L. M., Fagundes, C. P., & Butterworth, M. R. (2011). Attachment style, vagal tone, and empathy during mother–adolescent interactions. *Journal of Research on Adolescence, 22*(1), 165–184.

125 Grossman, P., Wilhelm, F. H., & Spoerle, M. (2004). Respiratory sinus arrhythmia, cardiac vagal control, and daily activity. *American Journal of Physiology, Heart and Circulatory Physiology, 287*(2), H728–734.

126 Taylor, M. J. (2003), cited in Dale, L. P., Carroll, L. E., Galen, G. C., Schein, R., et al. (2011). Yoga practice may buffer the deleterious effects of abuse on women's self-concept and dysfunctional coping. *Journal of Aggression, Maltreatment and Trauma, 20*(1), 90–102.

127 Sarang, P., & Telles, S. (2006). Effects of two yoga based relaxation techniques on heart rate variability (HRV). *International Journal of Stress Management, 13*(4), 460–475.

128 Khattab, K., Khattab, A. A., Ortak, J., Richardt, G., & Bonnemeier, H. (2007). Iyengar yoga increases cardiac parasympathetic nervous modulation among healthy yoga practitioners. *Evidence-Based Complementary and Alternative Medicine, 4*(4), 511–517.

129 Tyagi, A., Cohen, M., Reece, J., Telles, S., & Jones, L. (2016). Heart rate variability, flow, mood and mental stress during yoga practices in yoga practitioners, non-yoga practitioners and people with metabolic syndrome. *Applied Psychophysiology and Biofeedback, 41*(4), 381–393.

130 Breit, S., Kupferberg, A., Rogler, G., & Hasler, G. (2018). Vagus nerve as modulator of the brain–gut axis in psychiatric and inflammatory disorders. *Frontiers in Psychiatry, 9*, 44.

131 Coulter, D. (2004). *Anatomy of Hatha Yoga: A Manual for Students, Teachers, and Practitioners.* Honesdale, PA: Body and Breath.

132 Weiner, D., Weiner, P., & Beckerman, M. (2014). Anxiety dyspnea. *Harefuah, 153*(3–4), 147–50.

133 Porges, S. W. (2009). The polyvagal theory: New insights into adaptive reactions of the autonomic nervous system. *Cleveland Clinic Journal of Medicine, 76*(Suppl. 2), S86–S90.

134 Brown, R. P., & Gerbarg, P. L. (2005). Sudarshan Kriya yogic breathing in the treatment of stress, anxiety, and depression: Part I—Neurophysiologic model. *Journal of Alternative and Complementary Medicine, 11*, 189–201.

135 Jerath, R., Edry, J. W., Barnes, V. A., & Jerath, V. (2006). Physiology of long pranayamic breathing: Neural respiratory elements may provide a mechanism that explains how slow deep breathing shifts the autonomic nervous system. *Medical Hypotheses, 67*(3), 566–571.

136 Sullivan, M. B., Erb, M., Schmalzl, L., Moonaz, S., Noggle Taylor, J., & Porges, S. W. (2018). Yoga therapy and polyvagal theory: The convergence of traditional wisdom and contemporary neuroscience for self-regulation and resilience. *Frontiers in Human Neuroscience, 12*, 67.

137 Porges, S. W. (2009). The polyvagal theory: New insights into adaptive reactions of the autonomic nervous system. *Cleveland Clinic Journal of Medicine, 76*(Suppl. 2), S86–S90.

138 Jerath, R., Barnes, V. A., Dillard-Wright, D., Jerath, S., & Hamilton, B. (2012). Dynamic change of awareness during meditation techniques: Neural and physiological correlates. *Frontiers in Human Neuroscience, 6*, 131.

139 Pal, G. K., & Velkumary, S. (2004). Effect of short-term practice of breathing exercises on autonomic functions in normal human volunteers. *Indian Journal of Medical Research, 120*(2), 115–121.

140 Yadav, G., & Mutha, P. K. (2016). Deep breathing practice facilitates retention of newly learned motor skills. *Scientific Reports, 6*(1), 1–8.

141 Baghel, S. P., & Shamkuwar, S. S. (2017). Physiological review of qualitative impact of pranayama on respiration. *International Journal of Innovation and Research in Educational Sciences, 4*(1), 2349–5219.

142 Holloway & Ram (2004) and Benzo, R., Wigle, D., Novotny, P., Wetzstein, M. et al. (2012) cited in Barassi, G., Bellomo, R. G., Iulio, A. D., Lococo, A., et al. (2018). Pre-operative Rehabilitation in Lung Cancer Patients: Yoga Approach. In M. Pokorski (ed.) *Rehabilitation Science in Context*, pp. 19–29. Cham: Springer. p. .22.

143 Coulter, D. (2004). *Anatomy of Hatha Yoga: A Manual for Students, Teachers, and Practitioners.* Honesdale, PA: Body and Breath. p. 68.

144 Gosselink, R. (2003). Controlled breathing and dyspnea in patients with chronic obstructive pulmonary disease (COPD). *Journal of Rehabilitation Research and Development, 40*(5), 25–33.

145 Gilbert, C., Seals, D., Wyka, K., & Bradley, D. (1999). Breathing retraining: Advice from three therapists. *Journal of Bodywork and Movement Therapies, 3*(3), 159–167.

146 Pramanik, T., Pudasaini, B., & Prajapati, R. (2010). Immediate effect of a slow pace breathing exercise Bhramari pranayama on blood pressure and heart rate. *Nepal Medical College Journal, 12*(3), 154–157.

147 Serra, R. (2017). A Comparison of the Effects of Diaphragmatic Breathing Exercises and Yoga Pranayama Techniques on Pulmonary Function in Individuals with Exercise Induced Asthma. Unpublished thesis, Texas State University.

148 Liu, X. C., Pan, L., Hu, Q., Dong, W. P., Yan, J. H., & Dong, L. (2014). Effects of yoga training in patients with chronic obstructive pulmonary disease: A systematic review and meta-analysis. *Journal of Thoracic Disease, 6*(6), 795–802.

149 DeLuca, N. D., Vajta Gomez, J. P., Vital, I., Cahalin, L. P., & Campos, M. A. (2020). The impact of yoga on inspiratory muscle performance in veterans with COPD: A pilot study. *International Journal of Yoga Therapy, 31*(1), Article_4.

150 Nambinarayanan, T., Thakur, S., Krishnamurthy, N., & Chandrabose, A. (1992). Effect of yoga training on reaction time, respiratory endurance and muscle strength. *Indian Journal of Physiological Pharmacology, 36*(4), 229–233.

151 Nambinarayanan, T., Thakur, S., Krishnamurthy, N., & Chandrabose, A. (1992). Effect of yoga training on reaction time, respiratory endurance and muscle strength. *Indian Journal of Physiological Pharmacology, 36*(4), 229–233.

152 Mooventhan, A., & Khode, V. (2014). Effect of Bhramari pranayama and OM chanting on pulmonary function in healthy individuals: A prospective randomized control trial. *International Journal of Yoga, 7*(2), 104–110.

153 Anderson, B. E., & Bliven, K. C. H. (2017). The use of breathing exercises in the treatment of chronic, nonspecific low back pain. *Journal of Sport Rehabilitation, 26*(5), 452–458.

154 Mehling, W. E., Hamel, K. A., Acree, M., By, N., & Hecht, F. M. (2005). Randomized controlled trial of breath therapy for patients with chronic low back pain. *Alternative Therapies in Health and Medicine, 11*(4), 44–52.

155 Streeter, C. C., Gerbarg, P. L., Whitfield, T. H., Owen, L., et al. (2017). Treatment of major depressive disorder with Iyengar yoga and coherent breathing: A randomized controlled dosing study. *Journal of Alternative and Complementary Medicine, 23*(3), 201–207.

156 Cicek, S., & Basar, F. (2017). The effects of breathing techniques training on the duration of labor and anxiety levels of pregnant women. *Complementary Therapies in Clinical Practice, 29*, 213–219.

157 Obayashi, H., Urabe, Y., Yamanaka, Y., & Okuma, R. (2012). Effects of respiratory-muscle exercise on spinal curvature. *Journal of Sports Rehabilitation, 21*, 63–68.

158 Stephens, R. J., Haas, M., Moore, W. L., Emmil, J. R., Sipress, J. A., & Williams, A. (2017). Effects of diaphragmatic breathing patterns on balance: A preliminary clinical trial. *Journal of Manipulative and Physiological Therapeutics, 40*(3), 169–175.

159 Barros de Sa, R., Pessoa, M. F., Cavalcanti, A. G. L., Campos, S. L., et al. (2017). Immediate effects of respiratory muscle stretching on chest wall kinematic and electromyography in COPD patients. *Respiratory Physiology and Neurobiology, 242*, 1–7.

160 Sharma, V. K., Rajajeyakumar, M., Velkumary, S., Subramanian, S. K., et al. (2014). Effect of fast and slow pranayama practice on cognitive functions in healthy volunteers. *Journal of Clinical and Diagnostic Research: JCDR, 8*(1), 10–13.

161 Sharma, V. K., Rajajeyakumar, M., Velkumary, S., Subramanian, S. K., et al. (2014). Effect of fast and slow pranayama practice on cognitive functions in healthy volunteers. *Journal of Clinical and Diagnostic Research: JCDR, 8*(1), 10–13.

162 Anderson, B. E., & Bliven, K. C. H. (2017). The use of breathing exercises in the treatment of chronic, nonspecific low back pain. *Journal of Sport Rehabilitation*, *26*(5), 452–458.

163 Leahy, I., Schorpion, M., & Ganley, T. (2015). Common medial elbow injuries in the adolescent athlete. *Journal of Hand Therapy*, *28*(2), 201–210.

164 Bacchus, H. (2010). Breathwork and sports performance. *SportEX Dynamics*, *23*, 21–26.

165 Chatham, K., Baldwin, J., Griffiths, H., Summers, L., & Enright, S. (1999). Inspiratory muscle training improves shuttle run performance in healthy subjects. *Physiotherapy*, *85*(12), 676–683.

166 Bradley, H., & Esformes, J. D. (2014). Breathing pattern disorders and functional movement. *International Journal of Sports Physical Therapy*, *9*(1), 28–39.

167 Hodges, P. W., Butler, J. E., McKenzie, D. K., & Gandevia, S. C. (1997). Contraction of the human diaphragm during rapid postural adjustments. *Journal of Physiology*, *505*(2), 539–548.

168 Anderson, B. E., & Bliven, K. C. H. (2017). The use of breathing exercises in the treatment of chronic, nonspecific low back pain. *Journal of Sport Rehabilitation*, *26*(5), 452–458.

169 Perri, M. A., & Halford, E. (2004). Pain and faulty breathing: A pilot study. *Journal of Bodywork and Movement Therapies*, *8*(4), 297–306.

170 Pal, G. K., & Velkumary, S. (2004). Effect of short-term practice of breathing exercises on autonomic functions in normal human volunteers. *Indian Journal of Medical Research*, *120*(2), 115–121.

171 Jerath, R., & Barnes, V. A. (2009). Augmentation of mind-body therapy and role of deep slow breathing. *Journal of Complementary and Integrative Medicine*, *6*(1).

172 Jerath, R., Crawford, M. W., Barnes, V. A., & Harden, K. (2015). Self-regulation of breathing as a primary treatment for anxiety. *Applied Psychophysiology and Biofeedback*, *40*(2), 107–115.

173 Chalaye, P., Goffaux, P., Lafrenaye, S., & Marchand, S. (2009). Respiratory effects on experimental heat pain and cardiac activity. *Pain Medicine*, *10*(8), 1334–1340.

174 Ozgocmen, S., Cimen, O. B., & Ardicoglu, O. (2002). Relationship between chest expansion and respiratory muscle strength in patients with primary fibromyalgia. *Clinical Rheumatology*, *21*(1), 19–22.

175 Chapman, E. B., Hansen-Honeycutt, J., Nasypany, A., Baker, R. T., & May, J. (2016). A clinical guide to the assessment and treatment of breathing pattern disorders in the physically active: Part 1. *International Journal of Sports Physical Therapy*, *11*(5), 803–809.

176 Busch, V., Magerl, W., Kern, U., Haas, J., Hajak, G., & Eichhammer, P. (2012). The effect of deep and slow breathing on pain perception, autonomic activity, and mood processing—an experimental study. *Pain Medicine*, *13*(2), 215–228.

177 Jerath, R., Crawford, M. W., Barnes, V. A., & Harden, K. (2015). Self-regulation of breathing as a primary treatment for anxiety. *Applied Psychophysiology and Biofeedback*, *40*(2), 107–115.

178 Porges, S. W. (2003). The polyvagal theory: Phylogenetic contributions to social behavior. *Physiology and Behavior*, *79*(3), 503–513.

179 Porges, S. W. (2007). The polyvagal perspective. *Biological Psychology*, *74*(2), 116–143.

180 Porges, S. W. (2007). The polyvagal perspective. *Biological Psychology*, *74*(2), 116–143.

181 Garner, G. (2016). *Medical Therapeutic Yoga: Biopsychosocial Rehabilitation and Wellness Care*. Edinburgh: Handspring Publishing. pp. 45–46.

182 Garner, G. (2016). *Medical Therapeutic Yoga: Biopsychosocial Rehabilitation and Wellness Care*. Edinburgh: Handspring Publishing. p. 47.

183 Garner, G. (2016). *Medical Therapeutic Yoga: Biopsychosocial Rehabilitation and Wellness Care*. Edinburgh: Handspring Publishing. p. 47.

184 Streeter, C. C., Gerbarg, P. L., Saper, R. B., Ciraulo, D. A., & Brown, R. P. (2012). Effects of yoga on the autonomic nervous system, gamma-aminobutyric-acid, and allostasis in epilepsy, depression, and post-traumatic stress disorder. *Medical Hypotheses, 78*(5), 571–579.

185 Garner, G. (2016). *Medical Therapeutic Yoga: Biopsychosocial Rehabilitation and Wellness Care*. Edinburgh: Handspring Publishing. p. 46.

186 Bordoni, B., & Zanier, E. (2013). Anatomic connections of the diaphragm: Influence of respiration on the body system. *Journal of Multidisciplinary Healthcare, 6*, 281–291.

187 Prosko, S. (2019). Breathing and Pranayama in Pain Care. In N. Pearson, S. Prosko, & M. Sullivan (eds.) *Yoga and Science in Pain Care: Treating the Person in Pain* (pp. 141–157). London: Singing Dragon.

188 CliftonSmith, T., & Rowley, J. (2011). Breathing pattern disorders and physiotherapy: Inspiration for our profession. *Physical Therapy Reviews, 16*(1), 75–86.

189 Jerath, R., & Barnes, V. A. (2009). Augmentation of mind-body therapy and role of deep slow breathing. *Journal of Complementary and Integrative Medicine*. doi: 10.2202/1553-3840.1299.

190 Kaminoff, L. (2006). What yoga therapists should know about the anatomy of breathing. *International Journal of Yoga Therapy, 16*(1), 67–77.

191 Coulter, D. (2004). *Anatomy of Hatha Yoga: A Manual for Students, Teachers, and Practitioners*. Honesdale, PA: Body and Breath. p. 81.

192 Kaminoff, L. (2006). What yoga therapists should know about the anatomy of breathing. *International Journal of Yoga Therapy, 16*(1), 67–77.

193 Niehues, J. R. (2015). Pilates method for lung function and functional capacity in obese adults. *Alternative Therapies in Health and Medicine, 21*(5), 73–80.

194 Cobb, E. (2018, March 27). Episode 245: Band breathing is the new belly breathing. Z-Health. Accessed on August 18, 2019 at https://zhealtheducation.com/blog/band-breathing-is-the-new-belly-breathing.

195 Garner, G. (2016). *Medical Therapeutic Yoga: Biopsychosocial Rehabilitation and Wellness Care*. Edinburgh: Handspring Publishing.

196 Wiebe, J. (2015, December 2). *How Should You Breathe?* [Video file]. Accessed on August 19, 2018 at www.youtube.com/watch?v=Oj01gEJgEtk.

197 Schleifer, L. M., Ley, R., & Spalding, T. W. (2002). A hyperventilation theory of job stress and musculoskeletal disorders. *American Journal of Industrial Medicine, 41*(5), 420–432.

198 Berceli, D., & Napoli, M. (2007). A proposal for a mindfulness-based trauma prevention program for social work professionals. *Complementary Health Practice Review, 11*(3), 153–165.

199 Wang, M. Y., Greendale, G. A., Kazadi, L., & Salem, G. J. (2012). Yoga improves upper-extremity function and scapular posturing in persons with hyperkyphosis. *Journal of Yoga & Physical Therapy, 2*(3), 117.

200 Barassi, G., Bellomo, R. G., Iulio, A. D., Lococo, A., et al. (2018). Preoperative Rehabilitation in Lung Cancer Patients: Yoga Approach. In M. Pokorski (ed.) *Rehabilitation Science in Context*, pp. 19–29. Cham: Springer.

201 Barassi, G., Bellomo, R. G., Iulio, A. D., Lococo, A., et al. (2018). Preoperative Rehabilitation in Lung Cancer Patients: Yoga Approach. In M. Pokorski (ed.) *Rehabilitation Science in Context*, pp. 19–29. Cham: Springer. p. 22.

202 Brown, R. P., & Gerbarg, P. L. (2005). Sudarshan Kriya yogic breathing in the treatment of stress, anxiety, and depression: Part I—Neurophysiologic model. *Journal of Alternative and Complementary Medicine, 11*, 189–201.

203 Massery, M., Hagins, M., Stafford, R., Moerchen, V., & Hodges, P. W. (2013). Effect of airway control by glottal structures on postural stability. *Journal of Applied Physiology*, *115*(4), 483–490.

204 Massery, M. (2013, August 8). Soda pop can model—Massery PT—Mary Massery—If you can't breathe, you can't function [Video]. Massery PT. Accessed on January 4, 2023 at www.youtube.com/watch?v=leiKhMmjDGc.

205 Kumar, V., Malhotra, V., & Kumar, S. (2019). Application of standardised yoga protocols as the basis of physiotherapy recommendation in treatment of sleep apneas: Moving beyond pranayamas. *Indian Journal of Otolaryngology and Head and Neck Surgery*, *71*(1), 558–565.

206 Guimarães, K. C., Drager, L. F., Genta, P. R., Marcondes, B. F., & Lorenzi-Filho, G. (2009). Effects of oropharyngeal exercises on patients with moderate obstructive sleep apnea syndrome. *American Journal of Respiratory and Critical Care Medicine*, *179*(10), 962–966.

207 Erturk, N., Calik-Kutukcu, E., Arikan, H., Savci, S., et al. (2020). The effectiveness of oropharyngeal exercises compared to inspiratory muscle training in obstructive sleep apnea: A randomized controlled trial. *Heart & Lung*, *49*(6), 940–948.

208 Kumar, V., Malhotra, V., & Kumar, S. (2019). Application of standardised yoga protocols as the basis of physiotherapy recommendation in treatment of sleep apneas: Moving beyond pranayamas. *Indian Journal of Otolaryngology and Head and Neck Surgery*, *71*(1), 558–565.

209 Vernikos, J., Deepak, A., Sarkar, D. K., Rickards, C. A., & Convertino, V. A. (2012). Yoga therapy as a complement to astronaut health and emotional fitness—stress reduction and countermeasure effectiveness before, during, and in post-flight rehabilitation: A hypothesis. Accessed on January 4, 2023 at www.taksha.org/storage/2018/04/paper4.pdf.

210 Miles (1964), cited in Swami, G., Singh, S., Singh, K. P., & Gupta, M. (2010). Effect of yoga on pulmonary function tests of hypothyroid patients. *Indian Journal of Physiology and Pharmacology*, *54*(1), 51–56.

211 Hussein, N. A., Afify, A. M., Obaya, H. E., & Rafea, A. (2016). Effects of ujjayi pranayama training on selected ventilatory function test in patients with mild bronchial asthma. *Medical Journal of Cairo University*, *84*(2), 445–452.

212 Brown, R. P., & Gerberg, P. L. (2005). Sudarshan Kriya yogic breathing in the treatment of stress, anxiety, and depression: Part 1—Neurophysiologic model. *Journal of Alternative and Complementary Medicine*, *11*, 189–201.

213 Palkhivala, A. (2007, August 28). Aadil Palkhivala explains how to teach ujjayi breath. *Yoga Journal*. Accessed on June 3, 2022 at www.yogajournal.com/teach/teaching-methods/teaching-ujjayi-breath.

214 Park, H., & Han, D. (2015). The effect of the correlation between the contraction of the pelvic floor muscles and diaphragmatic motion during breathing. *Journal of Physical Therapy Science*, *27*(7), 2113–2115.

215 Cornwell, P., Ward, E., Lim, Y., & Wadsworth, B. (2014). Impact of an abdominal binder on speech outcomes in people with tetraplegic spinal cord injury: Perceptual and acoustic measures. *Topics in Spinal Cord Injury Rehabilitation*, *20*(1), 48–57.

216 Zolotow, N. (2022). *Yoga for Times of Change: Practices and Meditations for Moving Through Stress, Anxiety, Grief, and Life's Transitions*. Boulder, CO: Shambhala Publications.

217 Satchidananda, S. (1984). *The Yoga Sutras of Patanjali: Translation and Commentary by Sri Swami Satchidananda*. Yogaville, VA: Integral Yoga Publications. Sutra 2.3. p. 84.

Chapter 7

1 Burgin, T. (2022). The Cause of Suffering: The 5 Kleshas. Yoga Basics. Accessed on June 25, 2022 at www.yogabasics.com/learn/the-cause-of-suffering-the-kleshas.

2 Satchidananda, S. (1984). *The Yoga Sutras of Patanjali: Translation and Commentary by Sri Swami Satchidananda*. Yogaville, VA: Integral Yoga Publications. Sutra 2.3.

3 Wiech, K., & Tracey, I. (2009). The influence of negative emotions on pain: Behavioral effects and neural mechanisms. *Neuroimage*, *47*(3), 987–994.

4 Dale, L. P., Carroll, L. E., Galen, G. C., Schein, R., et al. (2011). Yoga practice may buffer the deleterious effects of abuse on women's self-concept and dysfunctional coping. *Journal of Aggression, Maltreatment and Trauma*, *20*(1), 90–102.

5 Sarang, P., & Telles, S. (2006). Effects of two yoga based relaxation techniques on heart rate variability (HRV). *International Journal of Stress Management*, *13*(4), 460–475.

6 Khattab, K., Khattab, A. A., Ortak, J., Richardt, G., & Bonnemeier, H. (2007). Iyengar yoga increases cardiac parasympathetic nervous modulation among healthy yoga practitioners. *Evidence-Based Complementary and Alternative Medicine*, *4*(4), 511–517.

7 Tyagi, A., Cohen, M., Reece, J., Telles, S., & Jones, L. (2016). Heart rate variability, flow, mood and mental stress during yoga practices in yoga practitioners, non-yoga practitioners and people with metabolic syndrome. *Applied Psychophysiology and Biofeedback*, *41*(4), 381–393.

8 Breit, S., Kupferberg, A., Rogler, G., & Hasler, G. (2018). Vagus nerve as modulator of the brain–gut axis in psychiatric and inflammatory disorders. *Frontiers in Psychiatry*, *9*, 44.

9 Joyce, C. T., Chernofsky, A., Lodi, S., Sherman, K. J., Saper, R. B., & Roseen, E. J. (2022). Do physical therapy and yoga improve pain and disability through psychological mechanisms? A causal mediation analysis of adults with chronic low back pain. *Journal of Orthopaedic and Sports Physical Therapy*, *52*(7), 470–483.

10 Joyce, C. T., Chernofsky, A., Lodi, S., Sherman, K. J., Saper, R. B., & Roseen, E. J. (2022). Do physical therapy and yoga improve pain and disability through psychological mechanisms? A causal mediation analysis of adults with chronic low back pain. *Journal of Orthopaedic and Sports Physical Therapy*, *52*(7), 470–483.

11 Ernst, G. (2017). Heart-rate variability—more than heart beats? *Frontiers in Public Health*, *5*, 240.

12 Sullivan, M. B., Erb, M., Schmalzl, L., Moonaz, S., Noggle Taylor, J., & Porges, S. W. (2018). Yoga therapy and polyvagal theory: The convergence of traditional wisdom and contemporary neuroscience for self-regulation and resilience. *Frontiers in Human Neuroscience*, *12*, 67.

13 Sullivan, M. B., Erb, M., Schmalzl, L., Moonaz, S., Noggle Taylor, J., & Porges, S. W. (2018). Yoga therapy and polyvagal theory: The convergence of traditional wisdom and contemporary neuroscience for self-regulation and resilience. *Frontiers in Human Neuroscience*, *12*, 67.

14 Sullivan, M. B., Erb, M., Schmalzl, L., Moonaz, S., Noggle Taylor, J., & Porges, S. W. (2018). Yoga therapy and polyvagal theory: The convergence of traditional wisdom and contemporary neuroscience for self-regulation and resilience. *Frontiers in Human Neuroscience*, *12*, 67.

15 Email conversation with Shelly Prosko, February 4, 2022.

16 Ernst, G. (2017). Heart-rate variability—more than heart beats? *Frontiers in Public Health*, *5*, 240.

17 International Association of Yoga Therapists (IAYT) (2012). Educational standards for the training of yoga therapists. Accessed on January 4, 2023 at www.iayt.org/page/ContemporaryDefiniti?&hhsearchterms=%22is+and+yoga+and+therapy%22.

18 Bhavanani, A. B., Sullivan, M., Taylor, M. J., & Wheeler, A. (2019). Shared foundations for practice: The language of yoga therapy. *Yoga Therapy Today*, *19*, 44–47.

19 Bhavanani, A. B., Sullivan, M., Taylor, M. J., & Wheeler, A. (2019). Shared foundations for practice: The language of yoga therapy. *Yoga Therapy Today*, *19*, 44–47.

20 Sullivan, M. B., Erb, M., Schmalzl, L., Moonaz, S., Noggle Taylor, J., & Porges, S. W. (2018). Yoga therapy and polyvagal theory: The convergence of traditional wisdom and contemporary neuroscience for self-regulation and resilience. *Frontiers in Human Neuroscience*, *12*, 67.

21 Sullivan, M. B., Erb, M., Schmalzl, L., Moonaz, S., Noggle Taylor, J., & Porges, S. W. (2018). Yoga therapy and polyvagal theory: The convergence of traditional wisdom and contemporary neuroscience for self-regulation and resilience. *Frontiers in Human Neuroscience*, *12*, 67.

22 Sullivan, M. B., Erb, M., Schmalzl, L., Moonaz, S., Noggle Taylor, J., & Porges, S. W. (2018). Yoga therapy and polyvagal theory: The convergence of traditional wisdom and contemporary neuroscience for self-regulation and resilience. *Frontiers in Human Neuroscience*, *12*, 67.

23 Sullivan, M. B., Moonaz, S., Weber, K., Taylor, J. N., & Schmalzl, L. (2018). Toward an explanatory framework for yoga therapy informed by philosophical and ethical perspectives. *Alternative Therapies in Health and Medicine*, *24*, 38–47.

24 Sullivan, M. B., Moonaz, S., Weber, K., Taylor, J. N., & Schmalzl, L. (2018). Toward an explanatory framework for yoga therapy informed by philosophical and ethical perspectives. *Alternative Therapies in Health and Medicine*, *24*, 38–47.

25 Sullivan, M. B., Moonaz, S., Weber, K., Taylor, J. N., & Schmalzl, L. (2018). Toward an explanatory framework for yoga therapy informed by philosophical and ethical perspectives. *Alternative Therapies in Health and Medicine*, *24*, 38–47.

26 Ray, U. S., Pathak, A., & Tomer, O. S. (2011). Hatha yoga practices: Energy expenditure, respiratory changes and intensity of exercise. *Evidence-Based Complementary and Alternative Medicine*. doi: 10.1093/ecam/neq046.

27 Streeter, C. C., Gerbarg, P. L., Saper, R. B., Ciraulo, D. A., & Brown, R. P. (2012). Effects of yoga on the autonomic nervous system, gamma-aminobutyric-acid, and allostasis in epilepsy, depression, and post-traumatic stress disorder. *Medical Hypotheses*, *78*(5), 571–579.

28 Streeter, C. C., Gerbarg, P. L., Saper, R. B., Ciraulo, D. A., & Brown, R. P. (2012). Effects of yoga on the autonomic nervous system, gamma-aminobutyric-acid, and allostasis in epilepsy, depression, and post-traumatic stress disorder. *Medical Hypotheses*, *78*(5), 571–579.

29 Sullivan, M. B., Erb, M., Schmalzl, L., Moonaz, S., Noggle Taylor, J., & Porges, S. W. (2018). Yoga therapy and polyvagal theory: The convergence of traditional wisdom and contemporary neuroscience for self-regulation and resilience. *Frontiers in Human Neuroscience*, *12*, 67.

30 Sullivan, M. B., Erb, M., Schmalzl, L., Moonaz, S., Noggle Taylor, J., & Porges, S. W. (2018). Yoga therapy and polyvagal theory: The convergence of traditional wisdom and contemporary neuroscience for self-regulation and resilience. *Frontiers in Human Neuroscience*, *12*, 67.

31 Guidi, J., Lucente, M., Sonino, N., & Fava, G. A. (2021). Allostatic load and its impact on health: A systematic review. *Psychotherapy and Psychosomatics*, *90*(1), 11–27.

32 Breit, S., Kupferberg, A., Rogler, G., & Hasler, G. (2018). Vagus nerve as modulator of the brain–gut axis in psychiatric and inflammatory disorders. *Frontiers in Psychiatry*, *9*, 44.

33 Schmalzl, L., & Sullivan, M. (2022). We know yoga works, but why? Mechanisms behind the practices' effects. *Yoga Therapy Today*. Accessed on June 22, 2022 at https://yogatherapy.health/wp-content/uploads/2022/05/YTT-Spring-2022_CE.pdf.

34 Cleveland Clinic (2021). Heart Rate Variability (HRV). Accessed on June 25, 2022 at https://my.clevelandclinic.org/health/symptoms/21773-heart-rate-variability-hrv.

35 Rollo, S., Tracey, J., & Prapavessis, H. (2017). Effects of a heart rate variability bio-feedback intervention on athletes psychological responses following injury: A pilot study. *International Journal of Sports Exercise Medicine, 3*(081), 1–14.

36 Aubert, A. E., Seps, B., & Beckers, F. (2003). Heart rate variability in athletes. *Sports Medicine, 33*(12), 889–919.

37 Karavidas, M. K., Lehrer, P. M., Vaschillo, E., Vaschillo, B., et al. (2007). Preliminary results of an open label study of heart rate variability biofeedback for the treatment of major depression. *Applied Psychophysiology and Biofeedback, 32*(1), 19–30.

38 Paul, M., & Garg, K. (2012). The effect of heart rate variability biofeedback on perfor-mance psychology of basketball players. *Applied Psychophysiology and Biofeedback, 37*, 131–144.

39 Muralikrishnan, K., Balakrishnan, B., Balasubramanian, K., & Visnegarawla, F. (2012). Cited in Nivethitha, L., Manjunath, N. K., & Mooventhan, A. (2017). Heart rate variability changes during and after the practice of bhramari pranayama. *International Journal of Yoga, 10*(2), 99–102.

40 Thayer, J. F., & Lane, R. D. (2009). Claude Bernard and the heart–brain connection: Further elaboration of a model of neurovisceral integration. *Neuroscience and Biobehavioral Reviews, 33*(2), 81–88.

41 McCraty, R. (2017). New frontiers in heart rate variability and social coherence research: Techniques, technologies, and implications for improving group dynam-ics and outcomes. *Frontiers in Public Health, 5*, 267.

42 McCraty, R., & Shaffer, F. (2015). Heart rate variability: New perspectives on physio-logical mechanisms, assessment of self-regulatory capacity, and health risk. *Global Advances in Health and Medicine, 4*(1), 46–61.

43 Cleveland Clinic (2021). Heart Rate Variability (HRV). Accessed on June 25, 2022 at https://my.clevelandclinic.org/health/symptoms/21773-heart-rate-variability-hrv.

44 Ernst, G. (2017). Heart-rate variability—more than heart beats? *Frontiers in Public Health, 5*, 240.

45 Ernst, G. (2017). Heart-rate variability—more than heart beats? *Frontiers in Public Health, 5*, 240.

46 Tyagi, A., & Cohen, M. (2016). Yoga and heart rate variability: A comprehensive review of the literature. *International Journal of Yoga, 9*, 97–113.

47 Telles, S., Sharma, S. K., & Balkrishna, A. (2014). Blood pressure and heart rate vari-ability during yoga-based alternate nostril breathing practice and breath awareness. *Medical Science Monitor Basic Research, 20*, 184–193.

48 Telles, S., Singh, N., & Balkrishna, A. (2011). Heart rate variability changes during high frequency yoga breathing and breath awareness. *Biopsychosocial Medicine, 5*, 4.

49 Nivethitha, L., Manjunath, N. K., & Mooventhan, A. (2017). Heart rate variability changes during and after the practice of bhramari pranayama. *International Journal of Yoga, 10*(2), 99–102.

50 Nivethitha, L., Manjunath, N. K., & Mooventhan, A. (2017). Heart rate variability changes during and after the practice of bhramari pranayama. *International Journal of Yoga, 10*(2), 99–102.

51 Schmalzl, L., & Sullivan, M. (2022). We know yoga works, but why? Mechanisms behind the practices' effects. *Yoga Therapy Today*. Accessed on June 22, 2022 at https://yogatherapy.health/wp-content/uploads/2022/05/YTT-Spring-2022_CE.pdf.

52 Schmalzl, L., & Sullivan, M. (2022). We know yoga works, but why? Mechanisms behind the practices' effects. *Yoga Therapy Today*. Accessed on June 22, 2022 at https://yogatherapy.health/wp-content/uploads/2022/05/YTT-Spring-2022_CE.pdf.

53 Schmalzl, L., & Sullivan, M. (2022). We know yoga works, but why? Mechanisms behind the practices' effects. *Yoga Therapy Today*. Accessed on June 22, 2022 at https://yogatherapy.health/wp-content/uploads/2022/05/YTT-Spring-2022_CE.pdf.

54 Sullivan, M. B., Erb, M., Schmalzl, L., Moonaz, S., Noggle Taylor, J., & Porges, S. W. (2018). Yoga therapy and polyvagal theory: The convergence of traditional wisdom and contemporary neuroscience for self-regulation and resilience. *Frontiers in Human Neuroscience, 12*, 67.

55 Rollo, S., Tracey, J., & Prapavessis, H. (2017). Effects of a heart rate variability biofeedback intervention on athletes psychological responses following injury: A pilot study. *International Journal of Sports Exercise Medicine, 3*(081), 1–14.

56 Physiopedia (2022). Vagus Nerve. Accessed on June 27, 2022 at www.physio-pedia.com/index.php?title=Vagus_Nerve&veaction=edit&section=9.

57 Physiopedia (2022). Vagus Nerve. Accessed on June 27, 2022 at www.physio-pedia.com/index.php?title=Vagus_Nerve&veaction=edit&section=9.

58 Bergland, C. (2014). How does the vagus nerve convey gut instincts to the brain? *Psychology Today*. Accessed on June 27, 2022 at www.psychologytoday.com/us/blog/the-athletes-way/201405/how-does-the-vagus-nerve-convey-gut-instincts-the-brain.

59 Physiopedia (2022). Gut Brain Axis (GBA). Accessed on July 1, 2022 at www.physio-pedia.com/Gut_Brain_Axis_(GBA).

60 Physiopedia (2022). Vagus Nerve. Accessed on June 27, 2022 at www.physio-pedia.com/index.php?title=Vagus_Nerve&veaction=edit&section=9.

61 Petra, A. I., Panagiotidou, S., Hatziagelaki, E., Stewart, J. M., Conti, P., & Theoharides, T. C. (2015). Gut-microbiota-brain axis and its effect on neuropsychiatric disorders with suspected immune dysregulation. *Clinical Therapeutics, 37*(5), 984–995.

62 Hadhazy, A. (2010, February 12). Think twice: How the gut's "second brain" influences mood and well-being. *Scientific American*. Accessed on November 29, 2022 at www.scientificamerican.com/article/gut-second-brain.

63 Radin, D. I., & Schlitz, M. J. (2005). Gut feelings, intuition and emotions: An exploratory study. *Journal of Alternative and Comprehensive Medicine, 11*(1), 85–91.

64 Naliboff, B. D., Berman, S., Suyenobu, B., Labus, J. S., et al. (2006). Longitudinal change in perceptual and brain activation response to visceral stimuli in irritable bowel syndrome patients. *Gastroenterology, 131*, 352–365.

65 Bonaz, B., Pellissier, S., Sinniger, V., Clarençon, D., Peinnequin, A., & Canini, F. (2012). The Irritable Bowel Syndrome: How Stress Can Affect the Amygdala Activity and the Brain-Gut Axis. In B. Ferry (ed.) *The Amygdala: A Discrete Multitasking Manager*. London: IntechOpen. doi: 10.5772/52066.

66 Labus, J. S., Mayer, E. A., Chang, L., Bolus, R., & Naliboff, B. D. (2007). The central role of gastrointestinal-specific anxiety in irritable bowel syndrome: Further validation of the visceral sensitivity index. *Psychosomatic Medicine, 69*, 89–98.

67 Merriam Webster (2022). Interoceptive [Definition]. Springfield, MA: Merriam Webster. Accessed on July 22, 2022 at www.merriam-webster.com/dictionary/interoceptive.

68 Paulus, M. P. (2013). The breathing conundrum—interoceptive sensitivity and anxiety. *Depression and Anxiety, 30*(4), 315–320.

69 Price, C. J., & Hooven, C. (2018). Interoceptive awareness skills for emotion regulation: Theory and approach of mindful awareness in body-oriented therapy (MABT). *Frontiers in Psychology, 9*, 798.

70 Garland, E. L. (2012). Pain processing in the human nervous system: A selective review of nociceptive and biobehavioral pathways. *Primary Care: Clinics in Office Practice, 39*(3), 561–571.

71 Khalsa, S. S., & Lapidus, R. C. (2016). Can interoception improve the pragmatic search for biomarkers in psychiatry? *Frontiers in Psychiatry, 7*, 121.

72 Craig, A. D. (2002). How do you feel? Interoception: The sense of the physiological condition of the body. *Nature Reviews Neuroscience, 3*(8), 655–666.

73 Paulus, M. P. (2013). The breathing conundrum—interoceptive sensitivity and anxiety. *Depression and Anxiety, 30*(4), 315–320.

74 Jafari, H., Courtois, I., Van den Bergh, O., Vlaeyen, J. W., & Van Diest, I. (2017). Pain and respiration: A systematic review. *Pain, 158*(6), 995–1006.

75 Herrero, J. L., Khuvis, S., Yeagle, E., Cerf, M., & Mehta, A. D. (2018). Breathing above the brain stem: Volitional control and attentional modulation in humans. *Journal of Neurophysiology, 119*(1), 145–159.

76 Ceunen, E., Vlaeyen, J. W., & Van Diest, I. (2016). On the origin of interoception. *Frontiers in Psychology, 7*, 743.

77 Armstrong, K. (2019, September 25). Interoception: How we understand our body's inner sensations. *APS Observer.* Accessed on November 29, 2022 at www.psychologicalscience.org/observer/interoception-how-we-understand-our-bodys-inner-sensations.

78 Price, C. J., & Hooven, C. (2018). Interoceptive awareness skills for emotion regulation: Theory and approach of mindful awareness in body-oriented therapy (MABT). *Frontiers in Psychology, 9*, 798.

79 US Department of Health and Human Services (2019). *Pain Management Best Practices Inter-Agency Task Force Report: Updates, Gaps, Inconsistencies, and Recommendations.* New York: US Department of Health and Human Services. Accessed on January 4, 2023 at www.hhs.gov/sites/default/files/pmtf-final-report-2019-05-23.pdf.

80 Kabat Zinn J. (2013), cited in McManus, C. (2017). Mindful awareness training: A promising treatment approach for persistent pain. *Pain Practitioner, 27*(1), 20–22.

81 Carlson, L. E. (2012). Mindfulness-based interventions for physical conditions: A narrative review evaluating levels of evidence. *International Scholarly Research Notices in Psychiatry.* doi: 10.5402/2012/651583.

82 Riegner, G., Posey, G., Oliva, V., Jung, Y., Mobley, W., & Zeidan, F. (2022). Disentangling self from pain: Mindfulness meditation-induced pain relief is driven by thalamic-default mode network decoupling. *Pain.* doi: 10.1097/j.pain.0000000000002731.

83 McManus, C. (2017). Mindful awareness training: A promising treatment approach for persistent pain. *Pain Practitioner, 27*(1), 20–22.

84 Riegner, G., Posey, G., Oliva, V., Jung, Y., Mobley, W., & Zeidan, F. (2022). Disentangling self from pain: Mindfulness meditation-induced pain relief is driven by thalamic-default mode network decoupling. *Pain.* doi: 10.1097/j.pain.0000000000002731.

85 McManus, C. (2017). Mindful awareness training: A promising treatment approach for persistent pain. *Pain Practitioner, 27*(1), 20–22.

86 Interagency Pain Research Coordinating Committee (2011). *National Pain Strategy Report.* Washington, DC: National Institute of Health. Accessed on July 9, 2022 at www.iprcc.nih.gov/node/5/national-pain-strategy-report.

87 Interagency Pain Research Coordinating Committee (2011). *National Pain Strategy Report.* Washington, DC: National Institute of Health. Accessed on July 9, 2022 at www.iprcc.nih.gov/node/5/national-pain-strategy-report.

88 Tatta, J., Willgens, A. M., & Palombaro, K. M. (2022). Mindfulness and acceptance-based interventions (MABIs) in physical therapist practice: The time is now. *Physical Therapy, 102*(3), pzab293.

89 Tatta, J., Willgens, A. M., & Palombaro, K. M. (2022). Mindfulness and acceptance-based interventions (MABIs) in physical therapist practice: The time is now.
Physical Therapy, 102(3), pzab293.

90 Kanter, G., Komesu, Y. M., Qaedan, F., Jeppson, P. C., et al. (2016). Mindfulness-based stress reduction as a novel treatment for interstitial cystitis/bladder
pain syndrome: A randomized controlled trial. *International Urogynecology Journal,
27*(11), 1705–1711.

91 Van Gordon, W., Shonin, E., & Griffiths, M. D. (2016). Meditation awareness training
for individuals with fibromyalgia syndrome: An interpretative phenomenological
analysis of participants' experiences. *Mindfulness, 7*(2), 409–419.

92 Adler-Neal, A. L., & Zeidan, F. (2017). Mindfulness meditation for fibromyalgia:
Mechanistic and clinical considerations. *Current Rheumatology Reports, 19*(9), 1–9.

93 Baker, J., Costa, D., & Nygaard, I. (2012). Mindfulness-based stress reduction for
treatment of urinary urge incontinence: A pilot study. *Female Pelvic Medical Reconstructive Surgery, 18*, 46–49.

94 Kearney, D. J. (2013). Loving-kindness meditation for posttraumatic stress disorder:
A pilot study. *Journal of Traumatic Stress, 26*, 426–434.

95 Kearney, D. J., McManus, C., Malte, C. A., Martinez, M. E., Felleman, B., & Simpson,
T. L. (2014). Loving-kindness meditation and the broaden-and-build theory of
positive emotions among veterans with posttraumatic stress disorder. *Medical
Care, 52*(12), S32–S38.

96 Fox, S. D., Flynn, E., & Allen, R. H. (2011). Mindfulness meditation for women with
chronic pelvic pain: A pilot study. *Journal of Reproductive Medicine, 56*(3–4), 158–162.

97 Doran, N. J. (2014). Experiencing wellness within illness: Exploring a mindfulness-based approach to chronic back pain. *Qualitative Health Research, 24*(6),
749–760.

98 Doran, N. J. (2014), cited in McManus, C. (2017). Mindful awareness training: A
promising treatment approach for persistent pain. *Pain Practitioner, 27*(1), 20–22.

99 McManus, C. (2012). Stress-induced hyperalgesia: Clinical implications for the
physical therapist. *Orthopedic Physical Therapy Practice, 24*(3), 165–168.

100 van Ravesteijn, H. J., Suijkerbuijk, Y. B., Langbroek, J. A., Muskens, E., et al. (2014).
Mindfulness-based cognitive therapy (MBCT) for patients with medically unexplained symptoms: Process of change. *Journal of Psychosomatic Research, 77*(1),
27–33.

101 Almonroeder, T. G., Kernozek, T., Cobb, S., Slavens, B., Wang, J., & Huddleston,
W. (2018). Cognitive demands influence lower extremity mechanics during a drop
vertical jump task in female athletes. *Journal of Orthopaedic and Sports Physical
Therapy, 48*(5), 381–387.

102 Paz, G. A., de Freitas Maia, M., Santana, H. G., Miranda, H., Lima, V., & Willson, J.
D. (2019). Knee frontal plane projection angle: A comparison study between drop
vertical jump and step-down tests with young volleyball athletes. *Journal of Sport
Rehabilitation, 28*(2), 153–158.

103 Almonroeder, T. G., Kernozek, T., Cobb, S., Slavens, B., Wang, J., & Huddleston,
W. (2018). Cognitive demands influence lower extremity mechanics during a drop
vertical jump task in female athletes. *Journal of Orthopaedic and Sports Physical
Therapy, 48*(5), 381–387.

104 Keeley, C. (2021). Conscious competence model and medicine. *Foot and Ankle
Surgery: Techniques, Reports & Cases, 1*(3), 100053.

105 McManus, C. (2017). Mindful awareness training: A promising treatment approach
for persistent pain. *Pain Practitioner, 27*(1), 20–22.

106 Niazi, A. K., & Niazi, S. K. (2011). Mindfulness-based stress reduction: A non-pharmacological approach for chronic illnesses. *North American Journal of Medical Sciences, 3*(1), 20–23.

107 Cherkin, D. C., Sherman, K. J., Balderson, B. H., Cook, A. J., et al. (2016). Effect of mindfulness-based stress reduction vs cognitive behavioral therapy or usual care on back pain and functional limitations in adults with chronic low back pain: A randomized clinical trial. *JAMA, 315*(12), 1240–1249.

108 Esch, T., Winkler, J., Auwärter, V., Gnann, H., Huber, R., & Schmidt, S. (2017). Neurobiological aspects of mindfulness in pain autoregulation: Unexpected results from a randomized-controlled trial and possible implications for meditation research. *Frontiers in Human Neuroscience, 10*, 674.

109 Russek, L., & McManus, C. (2015). A practical guide to integrating behavioral and psychologically informed approaches into physical therapist management of patients with chronic pain. *Orthopaedic Practice, 27*, 8–16.

110 Sullivan, M. B., Moonaz, S., Weber, K., Taylor, J. N., & Schmalzl, L. (2018). Toward an explanatory framework for yoga therapy informed by philosophical and ethical perspectives. *Alternative Therapies in Health and Medicine, 24*, 38–47.

111 Sullivan, M. B., Moonaz, S., Weber, K., Taylor, J. N., & Schmalzl, L. (2018). Toward an explanatory framework for yoga therapy informed by philosophical and ethical perspectives. *Alternative Therapies in Health and Medicine, 24*, 38–47.

112 Tonosu, J., Oka, H., Higashikawa, A., Okazaki, H., Tanaka, S., & Matsudaira, K. (2017). The associations between magnetic resonance imaging findings and low back pain: A 10-year longitudinal analysis. *PloS One, 12*(11), e0188057.

113 Kasch, R., Truthmann, J., Hancock, M. J., Maher, C. G., et al. (2022). Association of lumbar MRI findings with current and future back pain in a population-based cohort study. *Spine, 47*(3), 201–211.

114 Babińska, A., Wawrzynek, W., Czech, E., Skupiński, J., Szczygieł, J., & Łabuz-Roszak, B. (2019). No association between MRI changes in the lumbar spine and intensity of pain, quality of life, depressive and anxiety symptoms in patients with low back pain. *Neurologia i Neurochirurgia Polska, 53*(1), 74–82.

115 Vagaska, E., Litavcova, A., Srotova, I., Vlckova, E., et al. (2019). Do lumbar magnetic resonance imaging changes predict neuropathic pain in patients with chronic non-specific low back pain? *Medicine, 98*(17), e15377.

116 Ingraham, P. (2021, August 27). MRI and X-ray often worse than useless for back pain: Medical guidelines "strongly" discourage the use of MRI and X-ray in diagnosing low back pain, because they produce so many false alarms. PainScience. Accessed on October 15, 2022 at www.painscience.com/articles/mri-and-x-ray-almost-useless-for-back-pain.php.

117 El Barzouhi, A., Verwoerd, A. J., Peul, W. C., Verhagen, A. P., et al. (2016). Prognostic value of magnetic resonance imaging findings in patients with sciatica. *Journal of Neurosurgery: Spine, 24*(6), 978–985.

118 El Barzouhi, A., Verwoerd, A. J., Peul, W. C., Verhagen, A. P., et al. (2016). Prognostic value of magnetic resonance imaging findings in patients with sciatica. *Journal of Neurosurgery: Spine, 24*(6), 978–985.

119 Zoffness, R. (2019). A tale of two nails. *Psychology Today*. Accessed on July 9, 2022 at www.psychologytoday.com/us/blog/pain-explained/201911/tale-two-nails.

120 Zoffness, R. (2019). Think pain is purely medical? Think again. *Psychology Today*. Accessed on July 9, 2022 at www.psychologytoday.com/us/blog/pain-explained/201910/think-pain-is-purely-medical-think-again.

121 Louw, A., Farrell, K., Landers, M., Barclay, M., et al. (2017). The effect of manual therapy and neuroplasticity education on chronic low back pain: A randomized clinical trial. *Journal of Manual and Manipulative Therapy, 25*(5), 227–234.

122 Ashar, Y. K., Gordon, A., Schubiner, H., Uipi, C., et al. (2022). Effect of pain reprocessing therapy vs placebo and usual care for patients with chronic back pain: A randomized clinical trial. *JAMA Psychiatry, 79*, 13–23.

123 Zoffness, R. (2020). Research uncovers potential treatment for chronic pain. *Psychology Today*. Accessed on July 9, 2022 at www.psychologytoday.com/us/blog/pain-explained/202001/research-uncovers-potential-treatment-chronic-pain.

124 Desikachar, T. K. V. (1999). *The Heart of Yoga: Developing a Personal Practice*. New York: Simon and Schuster. p. 83.

125 Desikachar, T. K. V. (1999). *The Heart of Yoga: Developing a Personal Practice*. New York: Simon and Schuster. p. 83.

126 Desikachar, T. K. V. (1999). *The Heart of Yoga: Developing a Personal Practice*. New York: Simon and Schuster. p. 83.

127 Desikachar, T. K. V. (1999). *The Heart of Yoga: Developing a Personal Practice*. New York: Simon and Schuster. pp. 83–85.

128 Satchidananda, S. (1984). *The Yoga Sutras of Patanjali: Translation and Commentary by Sri Swami Satchidananda*. Yogaville, VA: Integral Yoga Publications. p. 100.

129 Satchidananda, S. (1984). *The Yoga Sutras of Patanjali: Translation and Commentary by Sri Swami Satchidananda*. Yogaville, VA: Integral Yoga Publications. p. 100.

130 O'Keeffe, M. (2016). *Treating More Than Just the Back: The Role of Individualised Multidimensional Care for Chronic Low Back Pain*. Doctoral thesis, University of Limerick, Ireland.

131 Hides, J., Donelson, R., Lee, D., Prather, H., Sahrmann, S., & Hodges, P. W. (2019). Convergence and divergence between exercise based approaches for management of low back pain that consider motor control. *Journal of Orthopaedic and Sports Physical Therapy, 49*, 437–452.

132 Sullivan, M. B., Erb, M., Schmalzl, L., Moonaz, S., Noggle Taylor, J., and Porges, S. W. (2018). Yoga therapy and polyvagal theory: The convergence of traditional wisdom and contemporary neuroscience for self-regulation and resilience. *Frontiers in Human Neuroscience, 12*, 67.

133 Sullivan, M. B., Erb, M., Schmalzl, L., Moonaz, S., Noggle Taylor, J., and Porges, S. W. (2018). Yoga therapy and polyvagal theory: The convergence of traditional wisdom and contemporary neuroscience for self-regulation and resilience. *Frontiers in Human Neuroscience, 12*, 67.

134 Desikachar, T. K. V. (1999). *The Heart of Yoga: Developing a Personal Practice*. New York: Simon and Schuster. p. 83.

135 Desikachar, T. K. V. (1999). *The Heart of Yoga: Developing a Personal Practice*. New York: Simon and Schuster.

136 Loizzo, J. J. (2016). The subtle body: An interoceptive map of central nervous system function and meditative mind-brain-body integration. *Annals of the New York Academy of Sciences, 1373*(1), 78–95.

137 Sullivan, M. B., Erb, M., Schmalzl, L., Moonaz, S., Noggle Taylor, J., and Porges, S. W. (2018). Yoga therapy and polyvagal theory: The convergence of traditional wisdom and contemporary neuroscience for self-regulation and resilience. *Frontiers in Human Neuroscience, 12*, 67.

138 Sullivan, M. (2019). Polyvagal Theory and the Gunas. In N. Pearson, S. Prosko, & M. Sullivan (eds.) *Yoga and Science in Pain Care: Treating the Person in Pain*, pp. 104–122. London: Singing Dragon. p. 114.

139 Sullivan, M. B., Erb, M., Schmalzl, L., Moonaz, S., Noggle Taylor, J., and Porges, S. W. (2018). Yoga therapy and polyvagal theory: The convergence of traditional wisdom and contemporary neuroscience for self-regulation and resilience. *Frontiers in Human Neuroscience, 12*, 67.

Chapter 8

1   Sparrowe, L. (2020, July 8). Understanding the gunas can help you find balance and insight. *Yoga Journal*. Accessed on August 5, 2022 at www.yogajournal.com/lifestyle/health/yoga-philosophy-101-3-gunas.
2   Sullivan, M. (2019). Polyvagal Theory and the Gunas. In N. Pearson, S. Prosko, & M. Sullivan (eds.) *Yoga and Science in Pain Care: Treating the Person in Pain* (pp. 104–122). London: Singing Dragon. p. 114.
3   Sovik, R. (2022). A Beginner's Guide to Bandhas. Yoga International. Accessed on June 5, 2022 at https://yogainternational.com/article/view/a-beginners-guide-to-bandhas.
4   Bhavanani, A. B., & Ramanathan, M. (2018). Psychophysiology of Yoga Postures: Ancient and Modern Perspectives of Asanas. In S. Telles & N. Singh (eds.) *Research-Based Perspectives on the Psychophysiology of Yoga* (pp. 1–16). Hershey, PA: IGI Global.
5   Chandaka, S., & Kandi, S. (2017). Yoga physiology and anatomy according to classical yoga and tantra texts. *Yoga, 2*(2), 365–368. Accessed on August 19, 2018 at www.theyogicjournal.com/pdf/2017/vol2issue2/PartG/2-2-58-482.pdf.
6   Chandaka, S., & Kandi, S. (2017). Yoga physiology and anatomy according to classical yoga and tantra texts. *Yoga, 2*(2), 365–368. Accessed on August 19, 2018 at www.theyogicjournal.com/pdf/2017/vol2issue2/PartG/2-2-58-482.pdf.
7   Chandaka, S., & Kandi, S. (2017). Yoga physiology and anatomy according to classical yoga and tantra texts. *Yoga, 2*(2), 365–368. Accessed on August 19, 2018 at www.theyogicjournal.com/pdf/2017/vol2issue2/PartG/2-2-58-482.pdf.
8   Iyengar, B. K. S. (1979). *Light on Yoga: Yoga Dipika*. New York: Schocken Books. pp. 379–380.
9   Gach, M. R. (1998). *Acu-Yoga: Self Help Techniques to Relieve Tension*. Uttar Pradesh: B. Jain Publishers. p. 61.
10 Gach, M. R. (1998). *Acu-Yoga: Self Help Techniques to Relieve Tension*. Uttar Pradesh: B. Jain Publishers. p. 61.
11 Gach, M. R. (1998). *Acu-Yoga: Self Help Techniques to Relieve Tension*. Uttar Pradesh: B. Jain Publishers. p. 61.
12 Iyengar, B. K. S. (1979). *Light on Yoga: Yoga Dipika*. New York: Schocken Books. p. 380.
13 Iyengar, B. K. S. (1979). *Light on Yoga: Yoga Dipika*. New York: Schocken Books. p. 439.
14 Iyengar, B. K. S. (1979). *Light on Yoga: Yoga Dipika*. New York: Schocken Books. pp. 439–440.
15 Burgin, T. (2019, October 1). The five vayus. Yoga Basics. Accessed on June 25, 2022 at www.yogabasics.com/learn/the-five-vayus.
16 Burgin, T. (2019, October 1). The five vayus. Yoga Basics. Accessed on June 25, 2022 at www.yogabasics.com/learn/the-five-vayus.
17 Burgin, T. (2019, October 1). The five vayus. Yoga Basics. Accessed on June 25, 2022 at www.yogabasics.com/learn/the-five-vayus.
18 Sovik, R. (2022). A Beginner's Guide to Bandhas. Yoga International. Accessed on June 5, 2022 at https://yogainternational.com/article/view/a-beginners-guide-to-bandhas.
19 Burgin, T. (2019, October 1). The five vayus. Yoga Basics. Accessed on June 25, 2022 at www.yogabasics.com/learn/the-five-vayus.
20 Burgin, T. (2019, October 1). The five vayus. Yoga Basics. Accessed on June 25, 2022 at www.yogabasics.com/learn/the-five-vayus.

21 Sovik, R. (2022). A Beginner's Guide to Bandhas. Yoga International. Accessed on June 5, 2022 at https://yogainternational.com/article/view/a-beginners-guide-to-bandhas.

22 Burgin, T. (2019, October 1). The five vayus. Yoga Basics. Accessed on June 25, 2022 at www.yogabasics.com/learn/the-five-vayus.

23 Sovik, R. (2022). A Beginner's Guide to Bandhas. Yoga International. Accessed on June 5, 2022 at https://yogainternational.com/article/view/a-beginners-guide-to-bandhas.

24 Burgin, T. (2019, October 1). The five vayus. Yoga Basics. Accessed on June 25, 2022 at www.yogabasics.com/learn/the-five-vayus.

25 Burgin, T. (2019, October 1). The five vayus. Yoga Basics. Accessed on June 25, 2022 at www.yogabasics.com/learn/the-five-vayus.

26 Sovik, R. (2022). A Beginner's Guide to Bandhas. Yoga International. Accessed on June 5, 2022 at https://yogainternational.com/article/view/a-beginners-guide-to-bandhas.

27 Burgin, T. (2019, October 1). The five vayus. Yoga Basics. Accessed on June 25, 2022 at www.yogabasics.com/learn/the-five-vayus.

28 Burgin, T. (2019, October 1). The five vayus. Yoga Basics. Accessed on June 25, 2022 at www.yogabasics.com/learn/the-five-vayus.

29 Burgin, T. (2019, October 1). The five vayus. Yoga Basics. Accessed on June 25, 2022 at www.yogabasics.com/learn/the-five-vayus.

30 Sovik, R. (2022). A Beginner's Guide to Bandhas. Yoga International. Accessed on June 5, 2022 at https://yogainternational.com/article/view/a-beginners-guide-to-bandhas.

31 Burgin, T. (2019, October 1). The five vayus. Yoga Basics. Accessed on June 25, 2022 at www.yogabasics.com/learn/the-five-vayus.

32 Sovik, R. (2022). A Beginner's Guide to Bandhas. Yoga International. Accessed on June 5, 2022 at https://yogainternational.com/article/view/a-beginners-guide-to-bandhas.

33 Coulter, D. (2004). *Anatomy of Hatha Yoga: A Manual for Students, Teachers, and Practitioners*. Honesdale, PA: Body and Breath. p. 177.

34 Coulter, D. (2004). *Anatomy of Hatha Yoga: A Manual for Students, Teachers, and Practitioners*. Honesdale, PA: Body and Breath. p. 177.

35 Coulter, D. (2004). *Anatomy of Hatha Yoga: A Manual for Students, Teachers, and Practitioners*. Honesdale, PA: Body and Breath. p. 177.

36 Desikachar, T. K. V. (1999). *The Heart of Yoga: Developing a Personal Practice.* New York: Simon and Schuster. p. 58.

37 Desikachar, T. K. V. (1999). *The Heart of Yoga: Developing a Personal Practice.* New York: Simon and Schuster. p. 58.

38 Hall, C., & Garden, S. (2022). Lost in Translation: Is Mulabandha Relevant for Modern Yogis? Yoga International. Accessed on June 18, 2019 at https://yogainternational.com/article/view/lost-in-translation-is-mulabandha-relevant-for-modern-yogis.

39 Coulter, D. (2004). *Anatomy of Hatha Yoga: A Manual for Students, Teachers, and Practitioners*. Honesdale, PA: Body and Breath. p. 158.

40 Coulter, D. (2004). *Anatomy of Hatha Yoga: A Manual for Students, Teachers, and Practitioners*. Honesdale, PA: Body and Breath. pp. 158–159.

41 Coulter, D. (2004). *Anatomy of Hatha Yoga: A Manual for Students, Teachers, and Practitioners*. Honesdale, PA: Body and Breath. pp. 204–205.

42 Coulter, D. (2004). *Anatomy of Hatha Yoga: A Manual for Students, Teachers, and Practitioners*. Honesdale, PA: Body and Breath.

43 Iyengar, B. K. S. (1979). *Light on Yoga: Yoga Dipika.* New York: Schocken Books.

44 Iyengar, B. K. S. (1979). *Light on Yoga: Yoga Dipika*. New York: Schocken Books. p. 436.

45 Mohan, A. G., & Mohan, I. (2004). *Yoga Therapy: A Guide to the Therapeutic Use of Yoga and Ayurveda for Health and Fitness*. Boston, MA: Shambhala. p. 135.

46 Vernikos, J., Deepak, A., Sarkar, D. K., Rickards, C. A., & Convertino, V. A. (2012). Yoga therapy as a complement to astronaut health and emotional fitness—stress reduction and countermeasure effectiveness before, during, and in post-flight rehabilitation: A hypothesis. Accessed on January 4, 2023 at www.taksha.org/storage/2018/04/paper4.pdf.

47 Mohan, A. G., & Mohan, I. (2004). *Yoga Therapy: A Guide to the Therapeutic Use of Yoga and Ayurveda for Health and Fitness*. Boston, MA: Shambhala. p. 135.

48 Mohan, A. G., & Mohan, I. (2004). *Yoga Therapy: A Guide to the Therapeutic Use of Yoga and Ayurveda for Health and Fitness*. Boston, MA: Shambhala. p. 135.

49 Vernikos, J., Deepak, A., Sarkar, D. K., Rickards, C. A., & Convertino, V. A. (2012). Yoga therapy as a complement to astronaut health and emotional fitness—stress reduction and countermeasure effectiveness before, during, and in post-flight rehabilitation: A hypothesis. Accessed on January 4, 2023 at www.taksha.org/storage/2018/04/paper4.pdf.

50 Mohan, A. G., & Mohan, I. (2004). *Yoga Therapy: A Guide to the Therapeutic Use of Yoga and Ayurveda for Health and Fitness*. Boston, MA: Shambhala. p. 135.

51 Desikachar, T. K. V. (1999). *The Heart of Yoga: Developing a Personal Practice*. New York: Simon and Schuster. p. 71.

52 Iyengar, B. K. S. (1979). *Light on Yoga: Yoga Dipika*. New York: Schocken Books. p. 436.

53 Iyengar, B. K. S. (1979). *Light on Yoga: Yoga Dipika*. New York: Schocken Books. p. 436.

54 Mohan, A. G., & Mohan, I. (2004). *Yoga Therapy: A Guide to the Therapeutic Use of Yoga and Ayurveda for Health and Fitness*. Boston, MA: Shambhala. p. 135.

55 Sovik, R. (2022). A Beginner's Guide to Bandhas. Yoga International. Accessed on June 5, 2022 at https://yogainternational.com/article/view/a-beginners-guide-to-bandhas.

56 Mohan, A. G., & Mohan, I. (2004). *Yoga Therapy: A Guide to the Therapeutic Use of Yoga and Ayurveda for Health and Fitness*. Boston, MA: Shambhala. p. 135.

57 Iyengar, B. K. S. (1979). *Light on Yoga: Yoga Dipika*. New York: Schocken Books. p. 438.

58 Mohan, A. G., & Mohan, I. (2004). *Yoga Therapy: A Guide to the Therapeutic Use of Yoga and Ayurveda for Health and Fitness*. Boston, MA: Shambhala. p. 135.

59 Kannan, P., Winser, S., Goonetilleke, R., & Cheing, G. (2018). Ankle positions potentially facilitating greater maximal contraction of pelvic floor muscles: A systematic review and meta-analysis. *Disability and Rehabilitation*, 1–9.

60 Coulter, D. (2004). *Anatomy of Hatha Yoga: A Manual for Students, Teachers, and Practitioners*. Honesdale, PA: Body and Breath.

61 Mohan, A. G., & Mohan, I. (2004). *Yoga Therapy: A Guide to the Therapeutic Use of Yoga and Ayurveda for Health and Fitness*. Boston, MA: Shambhala. p. 135.

62 Mohan, A. G., & Mohan, I. (2004). *Yoga Therapy: A Guide to the Therapeutic Use of Yoga and Ayurveda for Health and Fitness*. Boston, MA: Shambhala. p. 135.

63 Mohan, A. G., & Mohan, I. (2004). *Yoga Therapy: A Guide to the Therapeutic Use of Yoga and Ayurveda for Health and Fitness*. Boston, MA: Shambhala. p. 136.

64 Mohan, A. G., & Mohan, I. (2004). *Yoga Therapy: A Guide to the Therapeutic Use of Yoga and Ayurveda for Health and Fitness*. Boston, MA: Shambhala. p. 136.

65 Mohan, A. G., & Mohan, I. (2004). *Yoga Therapy: A Guide to the Therapeutic Use of Yoga and Ayurveda for Health and Fitness*. Boston, MA: Shambhala. p. 136.

66 Iyengar, B. K. S. (1979). *Light on Yoga: Yoga Dipika*. New York: Schocken Books. p. 147.

67 Kaminoff, L., & Matthews, A. (2012). *Yoga Anatomy*, 2nd edition. Champaign, IL: Human Kinetics. p. 28.

68 Desikachar, T. K. V. (1999). *The Heart of Yoga: Developing a Personal Practice*. New York: Simon and Schuster. p. 72.

69 Desikachar, T. K. V. (1999). *The Heart of Yoga: Developing a Personal Practice*. New York: Simon and Schuster. p. 73.

70 Desikachar, T. K. V. (1999). *The Heart of Yoga: Developing a Personal Practice*. New York: Simon and Schuster. p. 73.

71 Iyengar, B. K. S. (1979). *Light on Yoga: Yoga Dipika*. New York: Schocken Books. p. 148.

72 McDermott, D. (2023) IAYT Blog. How Yoga Therapy Works: Part 2—Frameworks for Understanding. Accessed on March 8, 2023 at https://yogatherapy.health/2023/02/09/how-yoga-therapy-works-part-2-frameworks-for-understanding.

Chapter 9

1 Altug, Z. (2021). Lifestyle medicine for chronic lower back pain: An evidence-based approach. *American Journal of Lifestyle Medicine, 15*(4), 425–433.

2 Fairbank, R. (2022, February 25). How simple exercises may save your lower back. *New York Times*. Accessed on March 4, 2022 at www.nytimes.com/2022/02/25/well/move/back-pain-exercises.html?.

3 Zoffness, R. (2020). Ten evidence-based strategies for pain relief. *Psychology Today*. Accessed on September 10, 2022 at www.psychologytoday.com/us/blog/pain-explained/202002/ten-evidence-based-strategies-pain-relief.

4 Goldish, G. D., Quast, J. E., Blow, J. J., & Kuskowski, M. A. (1994). Postural effects on intra-abdominal pressure during Valsalva maneuver. *Archives of Physical Medicine and Rehabilitation, 75*(3), 324–327.

5 Spencer, S., Wolf, A., & Rushton, A. (2016). Spinal-exercise prescription in sport: Classifying physical training and rehabilitation by intention and outcome. *Journal of Athletic Training, 51*(8), 613–628.

6 Almeida, M. B. A., Barra, A. A., Saltiel, F., Silva-Filho, A. L., Fonseca, A. M. R. M., & Figueiredo, E. M. (2016). Urinary incontinence and other pelvic floor dysfunctions in female athletes in Brazil: A cross-sectional study. *Scandinavian Journal of Medicine and Science in Sports, 26*(9), 1109–1116.

7 High, R., Thai, K., Virani, H., Kuehl, T., & Danford, J. (2020). Prevalence of pelvic floor disorders in female CrossFit athletes. *Female Pelvic Medicine and Reconstructive Surgery, 26*(8), 498–502.

8 Forner, L. B., Beckman, E. M., & Smith, M. D. (2020). Symptoms of pelvic organ prolapse in women who lift heavy weights for exercise: A cross-sectional survey. *International Urogynecology Journal, 31*(8), 1551–1558.

9 Wiebe, J. (2022, July 24). Weight Training and Prolapse—Is It OK? Accessed on September 10, 2022 at www.juliewiebept.com/weight-training-and-prolapse.

10 Wiebe, J. (2022, July 24). Weight Training and Prolapse—Is It OK? Accessed on September 10, 2022 at www.juliewiebept.com/weight-training-and-prolapse.

Chapter 10

1 Cronkleton, E. (2022). What Are the Benefits and Risks of Alternate Nostril Breathing? Healthline. Accessed on September 10, 2022 at www.healthline.com/health/alternate-nostril-breathing.

Chapter 11

1 Ishida, H., Hirose, R., & Watanabe, S. (2012). Comparison of changes in the contraction of the lateral abdominal muscles between the abdominal drawing-in maneuver and breath held at the maximum expiratory level. *Manual Therapy*, *17*(5), 427–431.

2 Chan, E. W. M., Hamid, M. S. A., Nadzalan, A. M., & Hafiz, E. (2020). Abdominal muscle activation: An EMG study of the Sahrmann five-level core stability test. *Hong Kong Physiotherapy Journal*, *40*(2), 89–97.

Index